RN Health Coaching

Manual For Success

Dwayne Adams, RN, MS

ISBN 978-0-9850033-6-4

ISBN 978-0-9850033-6-4

Legal Information & Disclaimers:

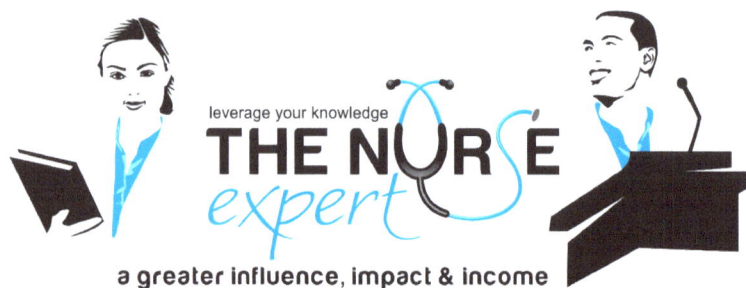

leverage your knowledge
THE NURSE expert
a greater influence, impact & income

www.TheNurseExpert.com

CONTENTS

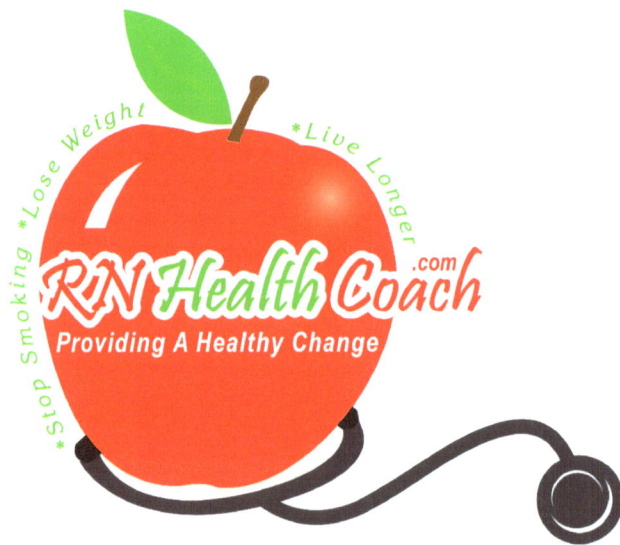

www.RNHealthCoach.com

Introduction

Respiratory diseases, cancer, diabetes and obesity, heart and liver disease and some psychological problems such as depression, are all strongly linked to health behavior, and lifestyle - and your doctor could not provide you a prescription for this, until now! Welcome the RN Health Coach as a solution. The above-mentioned diseases are largely preventable or remediable through Health Coaching and lifestyle change.

Mission:

To provide adequate resources allowing nurses to run, market and deliver an exemplary wellness program with a focus on weight management that will provide education, motivation and incentives to reduce the modifiable risks associated with weight-related health complications.

The Problem:

- Despite being **the largest spender on healthcare**, the U.S. has one of the **lowest life expectancies** of 77.9 years, according to the *United Nation's population division report*.
- Current health care is designed for the sick or diseased, **with little emphasis on prevention**.
- Healthcare **costs are 75% higher in overweight groups** compared to healthy weight groups.

You can be a solution:

- You possess the knowledge and experience.
- You are seen as an authority figure.
- You want to make a difference.

Why Focus on Weight loss?

Although your services are not limited to weight loss, we recognize being overweight as a causative agent to many medical health problems and conditions such as diabetes, hypertension, high cholesterol and heart disease, just to name a few. So the logic is, if we can help people achieve a healthy weight, we can limit the many other health hazards that exist as a result. Obesity is the second leading cause of preventable death. Tobacco is the first and we provide a solution for both! Be proud of yourself as an RN Health Coach, a soldier in this battle.

Do we stand a chance?

Yes, we do! Behavior can be modified. People can learn to take better care of themselves. Think of the example of smoking. Many groups of people in the United States have markedly decreased smoking. Of course there is still more work to be done. But if we can get some people to stop smoking, we can also help them learn to be healthy and lose weight.[1]

Why Does Coaching work?

Coaching is participant driven.

It provides accountability.

It is motivational for the participant.

70 to 80 percent of chronic disease is related to bad health behaviors, and lifestyle choices that we have control over.

Coaching works because of the synergy resulting from a professional partnership between the coach and the client.

RN Health Coaching: New Future, Major Need

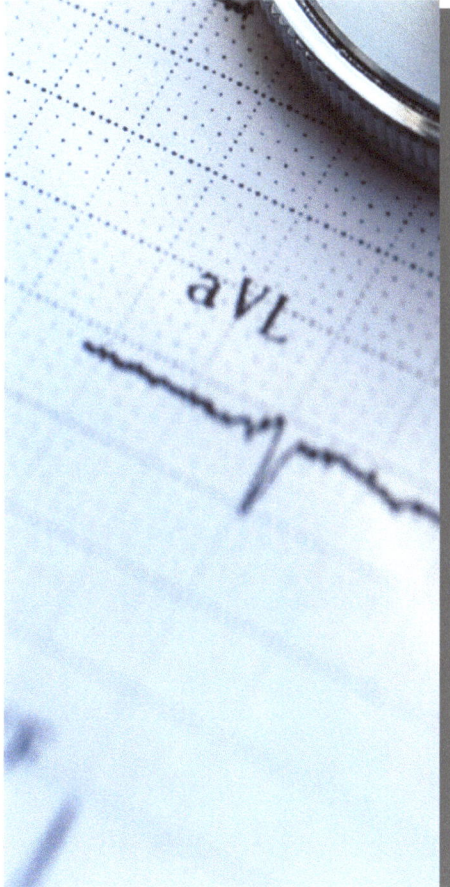

"Nursing in 10 or 20 years will look nothing like the nursing of today. New technologies and new drugs, changes in public attitudes toward health care and a shrinking workforce will force the profession to remake itself, probably several times over."

— NurseWeek Magazine: The Future of Nursing (2002)[i]

The combination of rising health care costs, insurance regulations and the increasing health needs of the aging baby boomers will work together to change the face and future of nursing. Many nurses fear the coming changes.

RN Health Coaching offers an opportunity to carve out the independence, financial freedom and entrepreneurial adventure of working for oneself.

The growing population of overweight and obese adults and the alarming indications of the rampant rise in childhood obesity point to the need for serious, medical solutions for the weight loss industry.

7

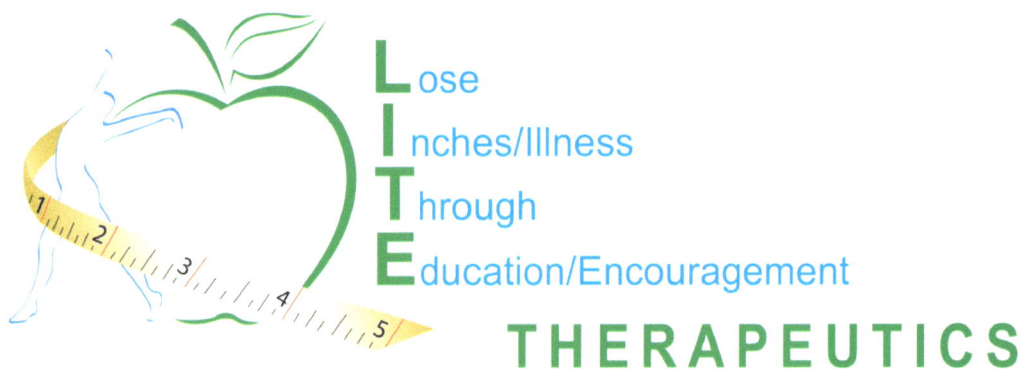

LITE

Lose
Inches/Illness
Through
Education/Encouragement

THERAPEUTICS

www.RNHealthCoach.com

www.HealthCoachNursingJobs.com

www.TheNurseExpert.com

The Need: Obesity, Being Overweight, Bad Habits & Looking for Real Solutions

Obesity and related conditions have grown at an alarming rate worldwide:

- The World Health Organization estimates that by 2015, 2.3 billion people will be overweight worldwide and more than 700 million will be obese.[ii]

- Estimates of the costs related to obesity and being overweight in the US by 2002 were $132 billion.[iii] *Ibid*.

- At the current trends the costs for obesity, being overweight and related problems in the US are projected to be $956.9 billion by the year 2030, making them an estimated 16-18% of the total US health care costs.[iv]

- People with a BMI over 45 (severely obese) live up to 20 years less than people who are not overweight.[v]

- 300,000 people die in the US annually from obesity and overweight health-related conditions.[vi]

In a desperate search for solutions, it is not unusual for the chronically overweight adult to try fad diets and extreme methods. The failure rate of this type of weight loss is estimated to be as high as 95%. On the other hand, we know that working with a weight-loss Health Coach significantly increases the success rate. *Bio-Medicine News*[vii]

The problem of achieving weight loss for so many people desperately needs to be addressed by nurses, with the skills, expertise and proven techniques that they provide. Health Coaching offers a tremendous opportunity to save lives, improve the quality of life and make a difference in the world.

RN Health Coach: A New Approach

An RN Health Counselor in Weight Loss is a personal advocate for making the right choices to live a healthy, energized life. Using a truly holistic approach to managing the weight loss process, all behavioral concerns are addressed including smoking, exercise and other life choices that impact weight and health; this includes managing the medical issues, spiritual and emotional issues as well.

RN Health Coach: A New Future

New trends in healthcare, changes in the management of hospitals and healthcare organizations have many nurses concerned about where their future will lead.

A RN Health Coach can determine his/her own hours, rates of pay and yearly income. The benefits and opportunities here are staggering. The ability to control work environment, hours and personal growth reduces the stress and anxiety of the job enormously.

The direct benefit of saving lives and improving the quality of life in one of the most serious medical conditions in the world is exciting.

This is a real chance to use your skills, expertise and personal commitment to make a meaningful change in the quality of health for many people in the world by addressing one of the fastest growing health concerns in the world.

Income Opportunity
Income Potential- Retire Your Current Job

There is an enormous amount of income that can be made after you gain the knowledge offered in this manual. As an RN Health Coach, you now have the opportunity to use your skill set in an environment never conceived of before. Imagine: the idea of receiving huge amounts of compensation from your own business while seeing clients outside of the hospital setting!

Yes it is possible. This opportunity can even allow you to retire as a bedside nurse.

Becoming a Health Coach RN offers so many career benefits and one of the most important is, without a doubt, how much income you can generate! Using your communication and clinical skills plus our unique program, you have in your hands the opportunity to build a business that meets your goals and provides for a secure and comfortable financial future.

Whether you are looking to augment your current income or wishing to become a full-time health coach, the amount of money you earn is up to you. Reaching the very pinnacle of the financial ladder is truly within your reach.

Let's look at a couple of scenarios when it comes to planning the income you wish to derive from your new career as a RN Health Coach.

In order to replace or realize an income of $50,000* per year, let's look at how many billable client-hours per week you would need to attain while charging different hourly rates:

Hourly Rate	Client Hours Per Week	Monthly Income
$50	21	$4200
$75	14	$4200
$100	10.5	$4200

*Registered Nurse Salaries — Staff RNs working in the United States average a median base salary of $41,642. Half of all US RN's are expected to earn between $38,792 and $44,869. Source: Allied Physicians — **Nurse Salaries & Nursing Salary Surveys**

Work More, Earn More   The Choice is Yours!

Now, take a look at the chart below for a representation of how your income can skyrocket based upon what you charge clients per hour combined with a *very reasonable* number of billable client-hours per week:

Hourly Rate	Client Hours Per Week	Monthly Income	Annual Income
$50	35	$7000	$84,000
$75	35	$10,500	$126,000
$100	35	$14,000	$168,000

Wellness Defined

Healthcare versus Wellness

Healthcare today is often viewed as reactive care. In fact, it is often seen as medical or sickness care. It is initiated after illness has stricken or you have a problem. This type of treatment is very expensive and much of the damage has already occurred. 99% of healthcare is reactive, while only 1% of government spending is on wellness or pro-active care, which lies on the opposite end of the health spectrum. While healthcare deals with death, disease and disability, wellness deals with optimum health through prevention and health promotion.

Currently, where does one go for wellness or proactive care? Few healthcare entities provide wellness care. This represents a prime opportunity for you as an RN Health Coach. The current system allows for many gaps in care. Often vital tests such as cholesterol levels are not conducted by doctors unless asked for. Who currently conducts a 360-degree review of your health? Because the individual has the most to gain from personal wellness, they have to take the responsibility for promoting it.

The Wellness Model

The National Wellness Institute has adopted the following definition of Wellness: "*Wellness is a process of becoming aware of and making choices toward a more successful existence.*"[viii]

Often weight loss efforts come after the weight has taken its toll on the client's life. Joints are damaged, diabetes has occurred, heart conditions are starting to impact the quality of life of the client.

The path from wellness to illness follows a series of signs, symptoms and disabilities prior to illness and premature death.

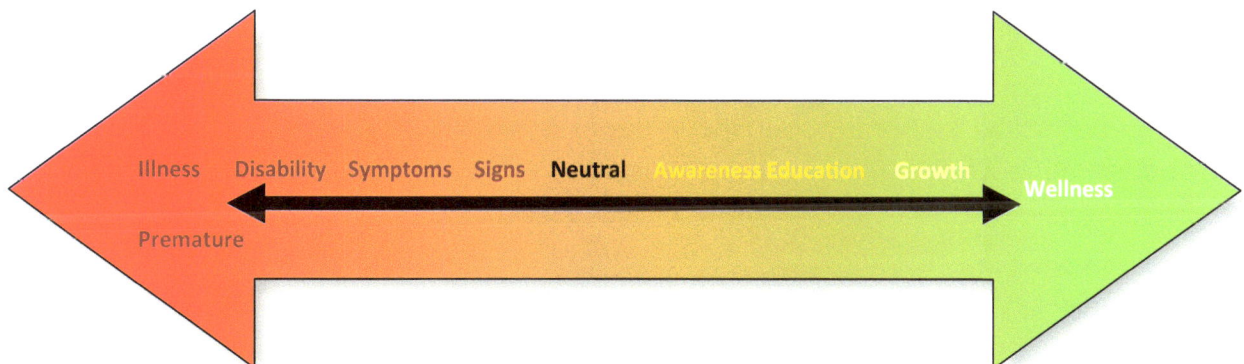

13

The most successful models for weight loss focus on awareness, education and growth rather than rapid reduction through strict dieting and strenuous exercise. Wellness models that embrace the complexity of weight loss will have the most success.

There are 6 major components to the wellness model shown below

1. Physical
2. Emotional
3. Intellectual
4. Social
5. Spiritual
6. Occupational

There is relationship within and among each component which needs to be addressed to create a strong model for success.

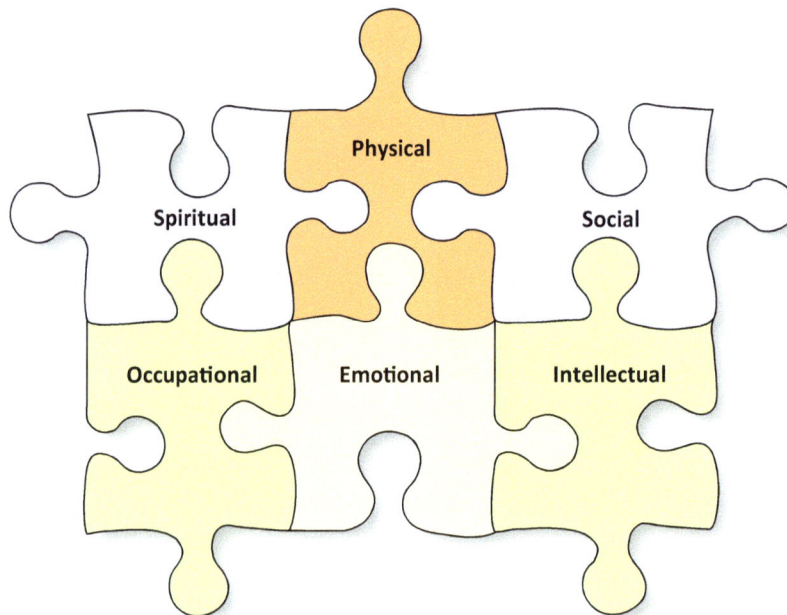

Often the components to wellness are hidden from the coaching environment. This model (shown below), often called the iceberg model, shows the complexity of what is visible compared to the interplay beneath the surface.

Spiritual/Meaning/Being Real

To make an impact in the weight of a client, an RN Health Coach must be able look at what they see in the coaching session, what they hear in the follow-up calls and what is underneath the discernable behaviors.

Travis' Iceberg Model of Wellness

Surface →

State of Health

Lifestyle: Behavioral Level

Cultural: Psychological and Motivational Levels

Spiritual/Meaning/Being Realm

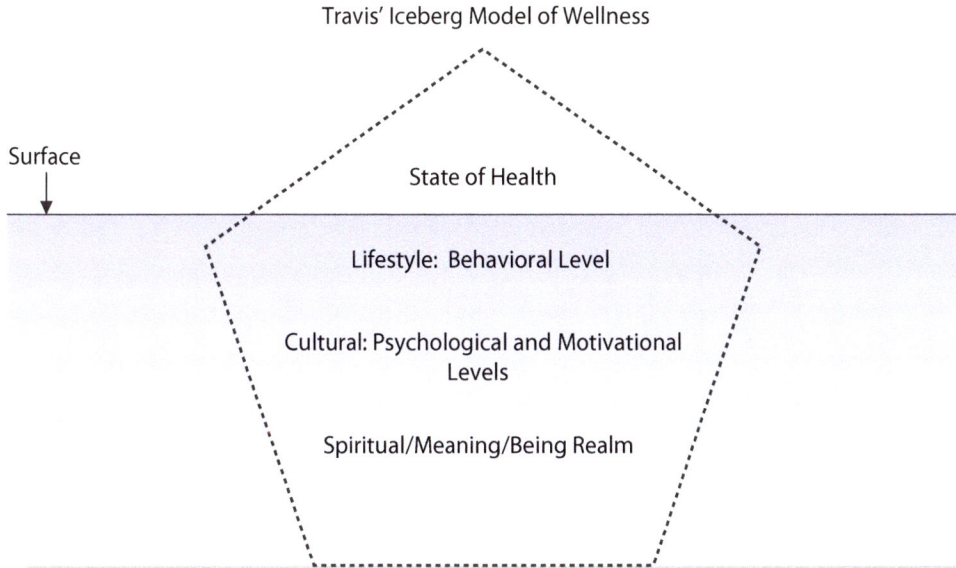

It is important to look at the client as a complex system and to focus as much on what is below the surface as on what is seen.

Often the habits and history of a client are masked in an attempt to seem less chronic; this can lead to difficulty in diagnosis and treatment.

Why Nurses make Perfect Health Coaches

Since education is a primary tenet of the nursing profession, the health coaching role is a natural. Coupled with the nurse's education in anatomy, physiology and general health issues, the health coach role seems to be crafted especially for nurses.

A nurse will be able to detect changes in signs and symptoms in the client, especially in related illnesses like diabetes and heart conditions as they related to weight loss.

Diagnostic training will be of strong benefit in the initial screening of the clients. Knowing what vital signs and measurements to take, and what conditions and medical history questions to ask about will aid in the understanding of the clients' issues both above and below the surface.

Since much of the follow up for the health coaching role is done remotely by phone, it is essential that the Health Coach have the ability to detect small changes, nonverbal indicators (like voice tone, pitch and volume) as a diagnostic aids to progress and process.

The client has more confidence in the Health Coach when they know that training, education and experience are there. In many health club roles, the trainer or diet consultant are hired for sales ability more than any degree or education.

15

This can create a dangerous scenario where a Health Coach could advise the client to do something outside of their health limits at the moment. Advising someone with joint issues from chronic obesity to jump rope, for example, would be a bad idea.

Prevention vs. Treatment

The RN Health Coach can create a preventative wellness program both for the individual and for a corporate organization. This focus on awareness, education and growth would allow both the individuals and the company to move toward wellness in a more holistic manner.

The LA Times, in an article in 2006, stated that Watson Wyatt Consulting Firm projected 54% of the largest US employers will offer health coaching to employees by 2007[ix]

The impact of wellness programs in reducing absenteeism, improving stress management and increasing productivity is so significant that most employers can justify the initial outlay because of the return on investment.

BB&T Corp. in Orlando finds that the wellness program has saved them on average more than $1000 per employee in health costs based on the industry averages.[x]

Co-existing Medical Conditions

Obesity increases the risk of developing one or more serious medical conditions leading to poor health and premature death. Obesity is linked to more than 30 medical conditions and at least 15 of those have been shown to have a strong link.

This includes the following conditions:

- Arthritis
- Cancers
- Cardiovascular Disease
- Sleep Apnea
- Deep Vein Thrombosis
- Diabetes
- End Stage Renal Disease
- Gallbladder Disease
- Hypertension
- Impaired Immune Response
- Impaired Respiratory Function
- Infections following Wounds
- Infertility
- Liver Disease
- Low Back Pain
- Obstetric and Gynecological Complications
- Pain

16

- Pancreatitis
- Stroke
- Surgical Complications
- Urinary Stress Incontinence

Weight loss of 10% of body weight can improve obesity-related conditions including diabetes and hypertension.[xi]

The RN Health Coach is the best choice for understanding the complexity of the conditions and how they impact the success of the weight-loss program.

17

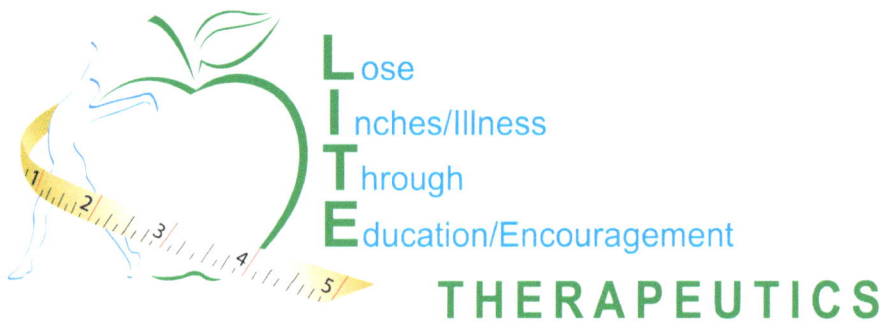

Lose
Inches/Illness
Through
Education/Encouragement

THERAPEUTICS

Coaching Fundamentals

RN Health Coaching Defined

The profession of health coaching is a merger of the worlds of psychology, training, business and counseling. The rapid increase in obesity has fueled the need for real solutions.

The Health Coach is at the heart a motivator, trying to inspire, encourage and enable clients to reach their goals. The unique qualifications of RN Health Coaches allow their vast experience, medical training and education to come together to facilitate the weight loss process for their clients.

Characteristics of a Good RN Health Coach

The health profession, like many helping industries, attracts a generous and giving population of professionals with good intentions and strong senses of purpose.

This niche of the market uses the power of persuasion, motivation and education to aid in the restructuring of behaviors, habits and lifestyles.

Dr. Michael Arloski, in his book "Wellness Coaching for Lasting Lifestyle Change," has identified the following 10 characteristics that describe a successful wellness coach:

- The coach needs to have a commitment to the healthiest lifestyle possible.
- The coach must have fairly low needs for control.
- The coach must be very centered emotionally and calm in a crisis.
- The coach must be patient but not indulgent or enabling with clients.
- A good coach will tend to see patterns and be a good system thinker.
- A coach needs to love to strategize and develop new ways to do things.
- A coach must believe that mind, body, spirit and environment all contribute to health and well-being.
- A coach must embrace challenges rather than fearing them.
- A coach should be perpetually curious about life in general and human behavior in particular.
- Coaches must be life-long learners.[xii]

Benefits of Health Coaching

Even under ideal conditions, weight loss is a difficult process. A lifetime of bad habits, little or no exercise, a sedentary lifestyle and the ever-increasing portion sizes of today's meals have created seriously adverse conditions to successful weight loss.

The difference an RN Health Coach makes is the significant factor of making sure the client is not alone in the fight. A coach, by definition, is there to craft the best possible results, strengthen the strengths and minimize the weaknesses, and to make the person accountable, responsible and successful.

One of the fundamental differences in coaching is that the process is more supportive than education or training.

In one study, the top 4 words associated with "COACHING" were: supportive, empowering, holistic and inspirational, while the words associated with "training" was prescriptive, rigid and intimidating.[xiii]

An RN Health Coach can aid the weight loss process in many ways including:

- Setting Goals.
- Identifying the barriers to weight loss.
- Educating the client about weight loss options.
- Encouraging and engaging physical activity.
- Empowering lifestyle changes.
- Breaking the daunting task down into manageable steps.
- Motivating the client to stay on track.
- Celebrating success.
- Providing accountability.
- Assisting with goal milestones.[xiv]

The combination of motivation, education, experience and role modeling a healthy and successful lifestyle, creates a collaborative process between the RN Health Coach and the client.

Personal benefits to being an RN Health Coach can include:

- Your personal development:
  o There is an old adage that says, if you want to learn something, teach it. The fastest way for a person to grow is to coach others.
- Income potential:
  o Coaching is a well-paid profession with a great deal of personal freedom in terms of where you work, how you work and how often you work.
- Building empowering relationships:
  o There is something transcendental about being the instrumental force in bettering another person's life. The connection in that process is enduring.
- Personal Mastery:
  o The call of this choice is to learn to be a role model for clients including living a life of wellness.
- Platform to Opportunity:
  o The skills that are learned, the growth during the experience, and the network created by coaching can lead to a wide range of opportunities, should the coach want to explore other opportunities.

- Give your Gift:
  - o Helping professions draw in people with an innate talent to care for and support others. If your gift is the ability to inspire, motivate and make a difference in someone's life, this is a wonderful stage for you.
- Be appreciated:
  - o In many jobs and careers, our hopes and aspirations get lost in the day-to-day experience of the job. This is a place where you can make a difference, save a life and be appreciated for the work you do.[xv]

Coaching: Therapy: Managing

The lines between coaching, therapy and managing can be a bit blurry. The RN Health Coach needs a strong understanding of the therapy process especially in the area of motivation and behavioral modification.

The management of the weight loss process will ultimately be in the hands of the client.

The role of the RN Health Coach assumes the client has the ability to be successful and that their role is to support the process. The RN Health Coach provides structure, support and tools to aid the success.

The process of being an ally in the fight on the side of the client changes the behaviors, assumptions and processes of the coach. The responsibility for change is the client's. The service becomes to work with the client, to partner the process and create an environment of support, collaboration and success.

Behavioral Change

The biggest hurdle to cross in order for weight loss to occur is to modify the lifetime of bad habits, false thinking and destructive internal dialogues that have led to the obesity. This is made difficult because of the sheer complexity of human behavior.

Whitworth, Kimsey-House and Sandahl in their book *Co-Active Coaching* identified four cornerstones for coaching.

1. Clients are naturally creative, resourceful and whole.

   Instead of approaching the client as someone needing fixing, approach them as whole and complete just as they are. Health conditions obviously can't be ignored but acceptance should be fundamental.

   This mindset on the part of the RN Health Coach creates a fostering environment where the client feels welcome, without judgment or condemnation.

2. Coaching addresses the clients' entire life.

   All the pieces in the puzzle fit together to impact the success or failure of the weight loss efforts; if there are tensions at work or problems at home they will impact the dedication, commitment and ultimately the success of the client.

21

The RN Health Coach needs to look at all the pieces in order to see the big picture come together.

3. The agenda comes from the client.

   The coaching model embraces the client-centered model; go where the client is and let them lead the process.

   Knowing where they are in the process shifts the mindset from prescriptive on the part of the Coach to facilitating and explorative.

4. The relationship is a designed alliance.[xvi]

   This is not a one-size-fits-all world. Every client will have different challenges and differing strengths. The Coach needs to be able to craft a unique environment for each client.

   The structure of the process, interviewing, measuring, and agreements may be the same but the client will add the complexity, the customization and the difference in the process.

Motivating Clients

Motivation is a well-researched discipline with loads of models for the causes and effects of motivation. The type of motivation (work, economic, wellness) can dictate the model. One of the enduring models of motivation is the work of Abraham Maslow from the sixties that is based upon the principles of deficiency and being.

Maslow's theory suggests that deficiencies are precedent in behaviors. At a basic level: food, water and air are deficiency needs. If they are not met we go beyond not functioning well to perishing.

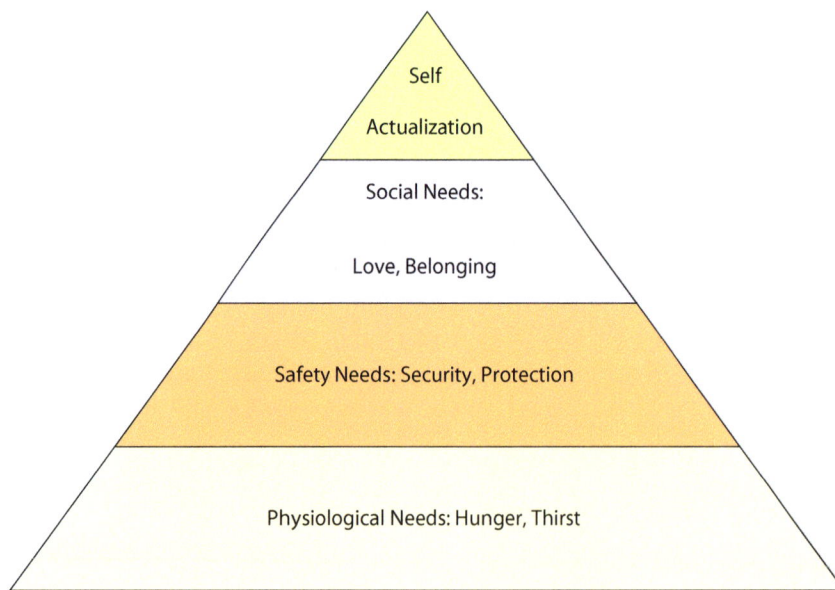

[i]

Self Actualization

Social Needs:

Love, Belonging

Safety Needs: Security, Protection

Physiological Needs: Hunger, Thirst

Maslow's Hierarchy of Needs[xvi]

22

In following the lifestyle of clients, it is clear to see them moving from level to level through the hierarchy. Coaching to wellness is an effective way of finding more efficient ways to meet needs at every level.

The "being" needs are more connected to realizing full potential as beings. Maslow believed that once deficiency needs were satisfied, we would seek personal growth. It is grounded in the belief that people are essentially good, and in the proper environment we will head to the "light."

Motivation is essential to the coaching process. Listening to the clients' stories and finding what barriers and obstacles have hindered their success in the past will provide insight into ways to motivate them through the daunting process of changing their lifestyle and managing their weight.

Finding the buttons that spark the desire in the client is a difficult process. Drawing on the diagnosis and triage practice is effective in peeling back the layers that protect real motivation, real desire and real incentive for the weight loss journey.

Bear in mind that the client may have a tremendous understanding of weight loss, as they may have been battling this all their lives. In many cases it is not from a lack of understanding, awareness or intellect but rather from an emotional or spiritual obstacle that they have yet to overcome. The more open, accepting and embracing the environment; the more likely the client is to share deeper layers of their history, and this awareness in both the client and the coach can lead to greater degrees of success.

For free training videos on how to become a RN Health Coach visit:

www.HealthCoachNursingJobs.com

Stages of change

We have the ability to change the following in life:

1. Our Behavior
2. Our Thoughts
3. Our Feelings

We can use the above to direct the goals we make.

In this section we will explore the 6 stages of change. Each stage calls for a different approach. You must know what stage you are in, so that the right tactic can be applied. Many other programs only address the action stage, which represents less than 20 percent of a problem population. Your knowledge of this will put you at a clear advantage.

Before we go into the 6 stages of change, let's explore what is called "The processes of change." There are nine:

1. Consciousness-raising
2. Social Liberation
3. Emotional arousal
4. Self re-evaluation
5. Commitment
6. Countering
7. Environment Control
8. Rewards
9. Helping Relationships

Let's explore each one in detail.

1. Consciousness Raising

"To make the unconscious conscious"

The goal of this process is to increase information about the problem and self. Raising one's level of awareness can improve the chance of making intelligent decisions.

2. Social Liberation
New alternatives can be given by the external environment. For example, no smoking areas, low fat menus.

3. Emotional arousal
Emotional arousal parallels consciousness raising, but on a more feeling level. It includes expressing and experiencing feelings about one's problems and solutions.

4. Self re-evaluation
Giving an emotional and thoughtful reappraisal of your problem and an assessment of the kind of person you will be once you have conquered the problem. "How do you perceive yourself as a sedentary person?" "How do you see yourself if you change your behavior?"

5. Commitment
Commitment means accepting responsibility for change. The first step is private; the second is public.

6. Countering and counter-conditioning
Countering means substituting alternatives for problem behaviors. For example, if a person tends to overeat when bored, he or she can replace or counter that by seeking out the company of a family member.

7. Environment control
This means avoiding stimuli that elicit problem behaviors. This is action oriented. Restructure your environment so that the probability of a problem-causing event is lowered.

8. Rewards
Reward yourself for making changes.

9. Helping Relationships
Find support or assistance from significant people in your life. Enlist the help of caring people.

26

Now let's dig into the 6 stages of change

Stage	Attitude
1. Pre-Contemplation	Never
2. Contemplation	Someday
3. Preparation	Soon
4. Action	Now
5. Maintenance	Forever
6. Relapse	

1. Pre-Contemplation

People in this group may often respond, "What problem?"

They or often unaware of a problem, not ready to change or haven't even thought about changing.

"It isn't that they can't see the solution. It is that they can't see the problem"

They lack information about their problem.

As a Health Coach, if you identify members in this stage, you can help by increasing awareness about change and the personal benefits that come along with making the change. As people become more aware of their problems, they become more receptive to help. Personalize information on risks and benefits. Talk about statistics, "Did you know...?"

"What would your life look like In 20 years if you don't stop...?"

"How does your behavior impact your spouse?"

Help start raising doubts.

Have the person:
- Make a list of benefits of change.
- Discuss need for change with someone they respect.
- Complete an HRA.

Tools to use:
- Posters
- Newsletters
- Awareness campaigns
- Policy
- HRA's
- Workplace Policies

27

- Screenings
- Advice from PMD
- Support groups

Process to use:
- Consciousness-Raising
- Social Liberation

Possible questions to ask in this stage include:

"What do people say to you about this behavior?"

"What would your life look like in 20 years if you don't stop smoking?"

The purpose is to help the client start to raise doubts.

2. Contemplation

Members in this stage are "waiting for the magic moment." They are thinking of making a change in the near future. They often feel stuck. They acknowledge that they have a problem, but have indefinite plans to change in the next 6 months.

As a Coach you should motivate and encourage making specific plans. Work to raise their consciousness.

"If you woke up tomorrow with all the courage in the world, what would you do?"

"If you had all the energy you need, what would you do?"

Evoke reasons from the client about why they may want to change.

Explore the risks of not changing.

Special technique:

1. **"Reflecting back the Challenge."**

    When a client describes a goal they are working on to you, reflect it back to them. Say, "Well, that sounds like hard work. Why would you invest so much energy?" This allows them to explore their reasons and help talk themselves into change.

2. **Use of Likert Scales.**

    For example: "On a scale of 1-10 - a 10 could be walking 5 times a week and 1 is not walking at all - where are you now?" Now it's time to explore. "Why did you give yourself that number? Why isn't it a lower number?" If they say six say "Why isn't it a seven?" or "Why did you give yourself a six?" Then say, "What would it take to increase from a six to an eight?" These are ways to help clients think about steps of moving into the preparation stage.

Have the person:
- Make a list of pros and cons.
- Talk to someone who made similar changes.

Tools to use:
- Posters
- Newsletters
- HRA's
- Workplace Policies
- Screenings
- Advice from PMD

Process to use:
- Consciousness-Raising
- Social Liberation
- Emotional Arousal
- Self Re-evaluation

3. Preparation

"I will soon." These members are making plans to change and are taking small steps. They might be making plans to get started within the next 30 days.

As a health coach, assist in developing an action plan and set gradual goals. You may assist in locating a class or support group. An important step is to make public the intension to change. "I will stop smoking on the 20th."
It is also necessary for you to help resolve any ambivalence.
Determine the best course of action in small steps.

The preparation stage is critical. Do not skip straight to action. This shortcut can actually lower their ultimate chance of success.

Good questions in this stage might be:
"What have you considered doing to get in better shape?"
"Would you like me to help you think through who might be a good exercise partner for you?"
"Would it be helpful if I helped you brainstorm on possible gym options in your neighborhood?" (You say it this way, instead of "Try such and such gym.")

Have the person:
- Write S.M.A.R.T. goals. (Specific, Measurable, Attainable, Relevant, Timely)
- Set rewards for reaching goals, non-food.
- Make a verbal commitment to those close to them. Make it public to the world.
- Research, read and find out what works best.
- Resolve ambivalence.

29

Tools to use:
- Directed self-study
- Self-care materials
- Awareness
- Health education events, lunches and learning opportunities.

Process to use:
- Social liberation
- Emotional Arousal
- Self Re-evaluation
- Commitment

4. Action

These people are ready to start now. Less than 20% or about 10-15% of people is in this stage at any given time. These people make a move for what they have been preparing for.

As a health coach you may assist with problem solving, provide support, help to refine goals. Have the member go public, tell others they are changing and why, and ask for support. Make plans for what to do in case of a relapse.

Tools to use:
- Health Coaching
- Directed self-study
- Support groups
- Contract

Process to use:
- Social liberation
- Commitment
- Reward
- Countering
- Environment Control
- Helping relationships

Provide encouragement and support in this stage. "What worked for you this week?" "What are you most proud of?"

Frame it as learning process. "What did you learn from that?"

5. Maintenance

These members plan to continue action.

30

Assist with reminders and avoiding relapse. Without a sure commitment to this maintenance stage, there will surely be relapse. This is a great opportunity to develop a maintenance plan for whatever coaching service you implement. For weight loss coaching you might remind them that millions of people have lost many pounds through different trendy diets, but regain the original weight.

Tools to use:
- Support groups (many coaches use and pay for TOPS for their clients)
- Tracking programs
- Incentive programs
- Telephone follow-up

Techniques to support behavioral change
- Goal setting
- Goal-related feedback
- Competition
- Rewards and incentives for goal achievement
- Contingency management

Process to use:
- Reward
- Countering
- Environment control
- Helping relationships

"How do you feel about what you have accomplished?" "What do you say to yourself about that accomplishment?"

Link accomplishment with values.

Honor success.

6. Relapse

Your members will experience relapses from time to time. It is important to let them know that this is natural, not to become discouraged. Most people try several times before they become permanently successful. As a coach you should not be judgmental or emotional. You will need to reevaluate their goals. Ask, "Where do you think we went wrong?" Try to plan a more achievable goal.

Help client debrief relapse.

Help normalize and reframe relapse.

Stay accountable yet avoid shame.

Re-link values.

Accessing Their Stage

One of your first steps should be to assess your client's stage of change. This can be easily done with just 4 questions. Ask the client whether or not they can say yes or no to the following statements:

1. I solved my problem more than six months ago.
2. I have taken action on my problem within the past six months.
3. I am intending to take action in the next month.
4. I am intending to take action in the next six months.

Question 1	No	No	No	No
Question 2	No	No	No	Yes
Question 3	No	No	Yes	N/A
Question 4	No	Yes	Yes	N/A
Your stage	**Pre-contemplation**	**Contemplation**	**Preparation**	**Action**

Compare their answers to this chart:

You have reached the maintenance stage when you can truthfully answer yes to statement 1. Coaches, now that you know the stage that your client is in you can begin applying tools from the appropriate 9 processes discussed earlier. Simple as that!

For ANY behavioral change, apply the BST Model

Behavior- Identify and agree on the behavior that needs to be changed.

Stage- Assess the stage of change your client is in by use of the 4 questions technique.

Tool- Apply the appropriate tools based on stage.

Now here is the chart once again with the Processes added.

Question 1	No	No	No	No
Question 2	No	No	No	Yes
Question 3	No	No	Yes	N/A
Question 4	No	Yes	Yes	N/A
Your stage	Precontemplation	Contemplation	Preparation	Action
Process to use	Consciousness-Raising, Social Liberation	Consciousness-Raising, Social Liberation, Emotional Arousal, Self-Re-evaluation	Social Liberation, Emotional arousal, Self-Re-evaluation Commitment	Social Liberation, Commitment, Reward, Countering, Environment Control, Helping Relationships

Motivational Interviewing

Motivational interviewing works by activating the client's own motivation for change and devotion to treatment. Your goal is to have *the client* say out loud *their* reasons to change. The style is "guiding" more than "directing," dancing rather than wrestling and listening more than telling.

"People are more persuaded by what they hear themselves say than by what someone else tells them" – Daryl J. Bem

The way you will elicit behavior change is based on Self-Perception Theory. This is the idea that change will occur if the client is the voice for change. The client should state the reasons for change and the process of change in order to become motivated. There is a huge difference between you telling clients what they should do for themselves and them saying what they should do for themselves. You as the coach will master the art of communication that allows the client to verbalize their change.

The essence/spirit of MI:

1. **Collaborative:** It is a partnership between you, the coach, and the client. It is an equal partnership, never about power

2. **Evocative:** Each client has their own personal goals, values, aspirations and dreams. Your goal is to connect behavior change with what your client cares about. As a coach you invoke their own good reasons and arguments for change. Activate the client's own motivation and resources for change. It is not about the nurse superimposing his or her wisdom or knowledge, or telling the client what to do. You should not even think that you have more wisdom or knowledge than they do.

3. **Honoring Client Autonomy:** You must have a certain degree of detachment from outcomes. The clients make the choice about the course of their lives. You may advise, inform or even warn, but ultimately it's up to the client.

Internalize the 3 above items and you will have Motivational Interviewing or Coaching Mastered.

Now that we talked about the spirit, let's discuss the RULES.

Four Guiding Principles: R.U.L.E.

1. **R-Resist the righting reflex.** It is natural tendency to fight persuasion, so don't "right" a client. If for example you say, "I think you are eating too much, and you should stop," the natural response is to argue the other side of the coin. "It's not that bad. I'm doing fine." Since we tend to believe

what we hear ourselves say, this would be counterproductive. The more the client verbalizes the disadvantage of change, the more committed they become to keeping the status quo. Give up the "having a problem" attitude.

2. **U-Understand clients' motivation.** It's the client's own reason for change, not yours! Ask the client why they would want to change and how they might do it, rather than telling them that they should.

3. **L-Listen.** Give up the attitude that you have all the answers and will inform the client. **When it comes to behavior change, the answer lies within the client**. Listen more than inform.

4. **Empower.** Outcomes are better when the clients take an active role in their care. Help them explore how they **can** make a difference in their own health.

Three Core Communication Styles

1. **Directing.** This type of style is familiar to you as a nurse. This is the telling or informing type of communication. It has a place, but very little in the coaching world. Try to limit this style.

2. **Following.** This is opposite of directing. You have no agenda. You are following where the client wants to go. You are a good listener.

3. **Guiding.** A guide helps you find your way. An example of guiding would be to listen empathically to understand a problem, and then ask for options they are considering. You both explore pros and cons of each together.

Three communication skills

1. Asking
2. Listening
3. Informing

Each of the above skills can be used in any style type.

1. Asking:
(Directing) "How many times has this happened?"
(Guiding) "What kind of change makes sense to you?"
(Following) "How have you been since the incident?"

2. Informing:
(Directing) "Your best option is to take these pills."
(Guiding) "Changing your diet would make sense medically, but how does that feel for you?"
(Following) "Yes, it's a common experience. Many clients also feel quite shocked and unsettled about simple things like going to the toilet"

3. Listening:

(Directing) "So you understand what's going to happen this morning, but you want me to tell you more about what will happen later on?"

34

(Guiding) "You're feeling concerned about your weight, and you are not sure where to go from here."
(Following) "This has been a huge shock."

1. Asking

Agenda Setting
There are many possible behavior changes a client could make to achieve their goal. A good coach will find out first where the client wants to go. The client sets the agenda.

"We are working on changing your diet. What would be most helpful for us to talk about today?"

Asking the right questions. The use of the "DARN" will be explained later.

Use a Ruler
Using a scale from 1 to 10 can tell you about a client's motivation, and also elicit change talk.
Step 1: Ask questions using the scale. "How strongly do you feel about eliminating excess sugar from your diet, where 1 is not strongly at all and 10 is very strongly?"
Step 2: Ask why they gave that number and not a lower number?
"Why did you give yourself a 7 and not a 3?"
The answer to this question is what we call "change talk." The client will talk themselves into changing (see next section).
Step 3: "What would it take for this number to go up?"

Pros and Cons
Asking pros and cons give you the opportunity to explore ambivalence.
First: Ask what is good about the way things are now. ***"What do you like about smoking?"*** This question elicits arguments for not changing.
Next: Ask about the not-so-good things regarding the status quo. ***"And what's the downside for you?"***
"What are the not-so-good things about smoking?" The answer to this question elicits "change talk."
Summarize this conversation with "Where does this leave you now?"

Key questions:
The essence of this question is "What next?" These are good questions to ask following the DARN techniques, ruler or pros and cons. The answer to these will activate commitment language.

- "So, what do you make of all of this now?"
- "What do you think you'll do?"
- "What would be a first step for you?"
- "What do you intend to do?"

Using Hypotheticals
The use of hypothetical language can make a client feel less threatened and allows greater freedom to envision change.

- "How would you like things to be different?"
- "Let's imagine for a moment that you did_____. How would your life be different?"

- "What might it take for you to make a decision to _____?"
- "If you did make a change in _____, what might be some benefits?"
- "If you were in my shoes, what advice would you give yourself about_____?"
- "How has (this behavior) kept you from growing, from moving forward?"

2. Listening

Taking the time to listen can result in making the client feel as though you spent a longer time with them than you actually have.

Make reflective listening statements

You can show that you are listening by reflecting a short summary of what is happening or what the client has said. Provide a short summary of how you understand what they said.

Provide a hypothesis about what the client means. Say it back in somewhat different words.

Try to offer at least two reflections for every question you ask.

Turn your questions into reflections:

1. Think of the question you want to ask.
2. Guess how the client might answer.
3. Say your answer out loud. Use a tone of voice like asking about the weather. Don't let the tone of your voice go up at the end.

3. Informing

Ask permission

Knock on the door before you open. Doing so honors and reinforces autonomy and active involvement in their care. It also displays the collaborative nature of your relationship as a coach and lowers resistance.

- "Would you like to know some things that other clients have done?"
- "Would it be ok if I tell you one concern I have about this plan?"
- "There are several things you can do to_____. Do you want to hear them, or are there other things we should discuss first?"
- "May I make a suggestion?"
- "You can tell me what you think of this idea..."

Offer choices

Don't tell your client what to do. Instead, offer choices. Offer a variety of options, and ask your client to choose among them. A rock-climbing guide using this philosophy might say, "If you look above you to the right, you will see that pointed rock, which could be unstable. One option is to reach up and try it. Another is to move over to you left, where you can stretch across to that ledge. Which move makes more sense to you?"

Talk about what others do

"Some clients in your situation reduce their intake of sugary foods. Others tackle their fat intake. I wonder what makes sense to you."

Be neutral. Provide information and let the client interpret.

Elicit-Provide-Elicit. EPE

1. Elicit

   "What would you most like to know about _____ (the information)?"

   "What do you already know about _____?"

2. Provide

   "Would you like for me to tell you a bit about_____?"

3. Elicit

   Ask open-ended questions to elicit responses to the information you provided.

   "What do you make of that?"

   "What does this mean for you?"

   "What more would you like to know?"

A good coach will:
- Ask where the client wants to go and get to know them a bit.
-Inform the person of options and see what makes sense to them.
-Listen to and respect what they want to do and offer help appropriately.

Why Won t A Client Change?

For the most part, people want to be healthy. They also already know some good reasons for behavior change that you have in your mind as a professional. They know they should exercise more, stop smoking, eat healthier, etc. You are not telling them anything new or what they don't know.

So what is the problem?

-Familiar routines.

-Unpleasant or painful feelings, such as lancing a finger for blood glucose, exercising after surgery, etc.

-Enjoyment of status quo.

The client has conflicting motivations. They have arguments on both sides (the good and bad associated with change). They are ambivalent. They know the good but understand it comes at an expense. They have reason to change, but they think of a reason not to change, then stop thinking about it altogether.

You are going to help your client talk themselves into change.

Things can happen to move a client toward or away from behavior change. An internal weighing of the pros and cons occurs, conscious or not. Think of your client as moving in one direction or the other, away from change, with cons or "resistance talk," or toward change, pros or "change talk."

The idea is to keep your client from talking "resistance talk" and encourage and evoke "change talk" or reasons from the client why they want to change. I will show you the technique soon.

I really want to emphasize this point about ambivalence. If you force only pro-change arguments on your client, the common response is to come back with the other side of the argument to say "Yes, but......" Then the client goes into resistance talk and reasons why they shouldn't, and talks themselves out of the change. Think about holding a baton. One end of the baton is "Yes I will do this," and the other end is "No, I will not do this." if you are holding the "Yes" side when you hand the baton to them, the only place they can take is "No" or in the middle. Stop pushing the yes side of the baton to the client. Hold the baton in the middle and hand it to the client so they can figure out which side they're going to land on.

Questions you don't want to ask:

-Why don't you want to_____?

-Why can't you _____ ?

-Why haven't you _____?

-Why do you need to _____?

-Why don't you _____?

These questions will elicit a response that is defensive and will reinforce the status quo.

Let s Talk Change. What is Change Talk?

There are six different types of change talk:

1. Desire
2. Ability
3. Reasons
4. Need
5. Commitment
6. Taking Steps

1. Desire
Verbs with the theme of desire include: **want, like,** and **wish**. These are statements about preference for change. Example: "I wish I could lose weight." "I like the idea of...."

2. Ability
Talk that reveals what a client perceives as within their ability. These are statements about capability. The verbs are **can** and **could**. Listen for "**might be able to**."

3. Reasons
Client expresses specific reasons for certain change.
"I would feel better if I exercised regularly."
"It would be good for my health."

4. Need

These include statements about feeling obliged to change. Key words are: **need, have to, got to, should, ought and must**.

5. Commitment

This includes statements about the likelihood of change.
I will, promise, guarantee, am ready to, intend to.

6. Taking Steps

These are statements about action taken. "This week I started…"
The client has done something that moves them in the direction of change.

Ok, Coaches: Here is how it works.

The first four types of "change talk" - desire, ability, reasons and need - are pre-commitment types. They can be remembered by the acronym DARN. Ask **DARN** questions followed by asking what steps would they take, and last, ask for the commitment. That was 3 steps. Here they go once again in detail:

1. Ask DARN questions

    A. "Why would you want to lose weight?" (Desire) "What do you want, like, wish, hope, etc."

    B. "How would you do it, if you decided to?" (Ability) "What is possible? What can or could you do? What are you able to do?"

    C. "What for you are the three best reasons for doing this?"(Reasons) "Why would you make this change? What would be some specific benefits? What risks would you like to decrease?"

    D. "How important is it for you to lose weight? (Need). "How important is this change? How much do you need to do it?"

2. Ask for steps

"What are you already doing to lose weight?" (Taking Steps)

3. Go for the commitment

"What do you think you would do?" (Commitment)

Evoke reasons from the client why they may want to change.

Explore the risks of not changing.

"People say that motivation doesn't last. Well, neither does bathing – that's why we recommend it daily." – Zig Ziglar

Summary of main points

- We are client centered.
- We are helping clients explore and resolve ambivalence.
- We let the client voice the argument for change.
- Talking about the change or behavior leads to believing in the change or behavior.

39

The Coaching Experience

Coaching Model

Coaching creates a synergy through the collaboration between the client and the coach. One of the critical steps in the process is to allow the client to have a voice in the process and to listen carefully to what they have to say.

Find Out What is Missing

There is a psychological belief that obesity is the result of trying to fill an emptiness that is totally unrelated to hunger. In listening to the client's story, listen for the clues about the elements of dissatisfaction, emptiness or need that may be holding the client back from success.

Assessment

The first session should include an intake interview to look for medical history, psychological issues or emotional challenges to the success of the project. Important physical parameters will be recorded such as BMI, Body Fat, Waist-to-Hip ratio, blood pressure, vitals, cholesterol and blood glucose to name a few. The interview is the time for the client to tell his or her story and this is place to begin to build the coaching relationship. Measurements and personal statistics are important to show progress, but the significant information will come from listening and powerful open-ended questions.

Goal Setting

Often the goals of clients are unrealistic and may lead them to feel as though they have failed. Discuss the goals with clarity and directness, and determine if the goals are practical. If a client needs to lose more than 100 pounds, the number can be daunting. Setting small goals can create a pattern of success rather than a pattern of failure.

Look Inside

Self esteem, personal value and boundaries are often related issues in obesity and poor lifestyle choices. A lifetime of reaching for food as comfort means that new problem-solving techniques and even new rewards need to be developed to facilitate success.

41

Environmental Factors

Routines and habits are best changed in an environment of support and structure. Help the client to establish a support network that is vested in their success. Look for related issues. Clutter is often a symptom of emotional distress; over-spending can also be an indicator of a life out of control. Does the client have other habits that will impede wellness? Does he or she smoke, drink excessively, or engage in other dangerous or unhealthy behaviors? Encourage your client to eliminate tempting foods from his or her environment at home and at work or school. Help the client develop a routine that will lead to positive changes in behavior.

Visualization

Create a strong vision in the clients' minds of what they will be like, feel like and live like as healthy people. For example: Keeping up with their children, traveling easily, moving swiftly or just being able to live a "normal" life without the drama that obesity may have brought them. For many chronically obese clients the simple things in life are out of reach. Can they use the bathtub? Fly on a commercial airplane? Drive a car? Ride on rides at an amusement park? Buy clothing easily? To have a clear vision in mind will aid the client through the difficult times in the process, will allow him or her to visualize success and will give the client an anchor in the process.

Fill the Gaps

Food journals, progress blogs or email reports all keep the relationship alive when the coach and the client are apart. The process will reinforce the lifestyle choices, heighten awareness, and will keep the client on track.

Bond Completely

Essential in this process is to create a strong initial bond. Often the first visit is done in the client's home, which allows the coach to have a sense of potential obstacles, challenges or support systems that may be in place. Initially, there may need to be more support or structure to cement that relationship. Over time, sessions may be conducted by phone with monthly following-ups in person.

Accountability

Part of the process is to hold the client responsible for the milestones, compliance with the process and appropriate effort. Be direct and challenge the client If the milestones are consistently not met.

Education

New techniques, new workout options or new menu planning ideas will all make the process easier for the clients. They may have standard coping mechanisms for diet and exercise that are built on years of failing, shame and guilt.

Providing new options and new techniques may provide the client with a new paradigm for success.

42

No Fear

Create a positive environment, without room for procrastination or excuses. When these problems occur, work to determine where the break in the resolve is coming from. Has stress increased at work, are there new problems at home or is there some old emotional dialogue that is preventing the success?

Empowering and Open-Ended Questions

The RN Health Coach needs to have a repertoire of open-ended questions that will encourage discussion, will allow the client to open up about fears and obstacles and will build new paradigms.

Open-Ended Questions might include:

- How did it go this week?
- What happens when you feel that way?
- What worries you most about the weight loss?
- Tell me more about your workouts this week
- What were you able to do?
- Why do you want to make this change?
- How important is this change?
- What are three of the most important benefits for you to successfully achieve your goals?
- What are you already doing to be healthy?

Yes and no questions do not open a dialogue. Open-ended questions lead to longer answers, more reflection and deeper insight for the coach.

Records and Charting Progress

The RN Health Coach needs to develop a set of intake and progress forms for tracking the process with the client. Careful collection of personal information (name, address, phone, email, etc), health history (diabetes, heart conditions, joint weakness or other factors important in the design of fitness and exercise routines) and goal-setting objectives are all essential information for building your practice.

Accounting records or commercial accounting software packages like Peachtree or QuickBooks can track the payment and balances for each client and make tax preparation for the business an easy process.

Files should be easy to find if the client contacts you outside of standard appointment times. Recording interventions, weekly targets and important elements of the dialogue will make the coaching process easier to follow and chart.

Charts and graphs can give visual impact to the tracking process, allowing the clients to see easily the progress they are making.

43

Even if the session is being conducted by phone the coach needs to maintain the ability to take notes, record information and gauge the mood, demeanor and emotional level of the client.

Coaching System

Create a contract template, a sample agreement and a policy and procedure document for each client, along with the standard accounting information forms to ensure payment.

This allows the coach to easily see where the client is in the process and also begins to build the "expert" view in the client's mind. The coaching system will create the structure and foundation for the coaching experience.

Business Models

As a business you will want to keep files, documents and records in a systematic fashion. You will need to file income for taxes, maintain an accounting system or use a professional accountant and schedule time appropriately. Since this is your business, you can control the processes. Create centralized forms that allow for the variation from client to client but creates a common structure or format.

Marketing Your Business

The Product. What am I selling?

The RN Coaching program focuses on **Weight Loss and Smoking Cessation**. We place a heavy emphasis on behavioral change techniques and motivational therapy.

Your services can be offered to the **general public** or to **small businesses** as a Wellness Program that you develop for their employees.

The services that you can offer are endless. You can specialize in wellness programs or on the other end, disease management. You can create any program for any population such as a:

- Cholesterol Reduction Program
- Defeating Diabetes Program
- Cancer Prevention Program

The names of the programs may differ but the process of motivating and delivering information to effect change is the same.

Some coaches even specialize in **speaking engagements** and **seminars**.

You can update the products you offer in your administrative section of the site. List your services and assign a fee to it all from your computer.

Price. What should I charge?

As the owner of your own coaching business you can charge any price you choose for your professional services. We recommend you price your programs according to the time it will take to deliver that program in its entirety. Charge clients for billable hours involved in delivering your program. Total up the amount of personal contact time, travel, phone calls, etc. Your minimum rate per hour should be no less than what you currently make as a Staff RN. We recommend anywhere in the range of $75-$100 dollars per hour. A few coaches earn up to $200 per hour. So, if you as a coach have a program which totals 2.5 hours of your time between visits and calls and your rate is $100/hour, you would charge $250 as a fee for this service. Bill for the hours it takes to deliver your program.

In addition to earning from your coaching services, we will give you $250 for every qualified referral that signs up with our RN Coaching program. The referral must utilize your email address when signing up. If your referral signs up using a sale or promotional price you will receive 50% of the fee instead of

45

$250. Your referrals can be traced in your admin area. This promotion is subject to change and may not last forever.

Prices for your products and services can be updated in your admin area of the site. You can bill your clients from this platform using Paypal.com

Position. How our services are different or unique

The ways we differentiate our services from typical weight loss services are as follows:

- Our services are delivered by professional, educated healthcare individuals vs. a lay person off the street.

- We place an emphasis on "coaching," motivation, and behavioral change strategies vs. directive "tell you what to do programs."

- We provide more than just weight loss advice - the client receives the benefits of your RN knowledge and can receive screenings for other health conditions and concerns.

You should ingrain in your head, how we stand out from the crowd. Visit these two sections of our website and internalize our differences:

http://rnhealthcoach.com/the_lite_philosophy.php

http://rnhealthcoach.com/comparison.php

Place. Where is my service delivered?

Your coaching service can be carried out in person, over the phone, internet or any combination. The following sites make it possible to deliver presentations over the net remotely with clients so they may view files that you have, such as PowerPoint presentations:

- www.gotomypc.com
- www.webex.cm
- www.webconference.com
- www.gotomeeting.com
- www.FreeConference.com

Promotion. How can I let prospects know about my service?

We are dedicated to assisting you with your marketing and promotion efforts. Think of us as your business coach. As a member, you can contact us with any questions or concerns you may have in respect to marketing your business and how we may assist you. We are continuously creating new marketing material for your needs. Be sure to check the free marketing section of your admin area for additions. We also have marketing tools for your purchase.

Below you will find the major ways to communicate your services as a coach.

Sales promotions

You can implement any special sales promotion you can think of and add it to your profile via your admin area. Visit this area of the site to update/list or edit the promotions you would like to list on your profile. Here is a list of some common or default promotions that you may choose to participate in:

- $50 back at the completion of your weight loss program. The dollars can be applied to an authorized purchase such as a gym membership, doctor's visit, and prescription medications. Advertisements can be placed at these facilities with their approval to alert the public of this great benefit. We will even create the ad for you! Just contact us.

- Spouse free, friends 50% off (up to 2 at the same meeting place).

- Any other promotions you can think of or wish to offer - just add it to your profile.

Strategic alliances

Contact your local gym, spa, pharmacy or doctors office **and work with them**. Offer them a percentage of sales, referrals or benefits to their clients for use and promotion of your services. Think win-win situation. We have created a great letter that you can send to local MD's in your area asking for referrals. **This one letter will do wonders for your business!** Check the marketing section of your site admin area. When approaching physicians, be aware of the fact that there may be differences between your approach to weight loss and their approach. Try to find common ground. Let the physician know you would like to work *with* him/her.

Public Relations

- Contact your local newspapers or magazines; send a letter expressing your desire to write a column or story for their paper. **Guess what**? That template letter is available to you in your free marketing section of your admin area. **That's not all!** If accepted by the paper, **we will write the articles for you!** That is a member benefit.

- Write a press release.

Online

Use online marketing to drive people to your profile page. Remember, your direct profile can be found at www.RNHealthCoach.com/"your_First_Name"/. You can always purchase your own domain name such as mycoachingbusinessname.com and point it (forward it) toward your designed profile page. As a member benefit, **we can take care of this process for you**.

You will want to use search term advertising in your *local area* to find people who are looking for your services and drive them to your site. Here are the websites you want to visit, listed in order of importance.

47

www.adwords.google.com

www.searchmarketing.yahoo.com

https://adcenter.microsoft.com

Once you have set up an account with the above site, you want to pick the appropriate key words such as:

- Health coaching, Health Coaches, Health Coach.
- Weight loss coaching, weight loss coach, health and wellness coach, wellness coach.
- Weight loss programs.
- Stop smoking programs, smoking cessation.
- Employee wellness programs.

Make sure your search term only attracts people in your local area. This is a special option you will have to choose. This will be a better use of your advertising funds as you provide the greatest benefits to those you can reach out to personally.

Direct Mail
Your marketing communications can be directed to:

- Potential clients of health coaching services
- Doctors
- Small business
- Spas

You can send postcards or letters. Postcards have the advantage of delivering your message immediately without the need to open a letter that might be discarded by the recipient. We can help you find brochures and letters, either free or for a small fee. We can also quote you on a mailing list with many criteria that will be sure to pinpoint your exact target market.

Fairs & Trade Shows
Be on the lookout for local health fairs. Participate in some manner in these events. This is a great way to make the public aware of your services and capture business.

Advertising
Radio - this may be a great way to advertise your service. In your Google adwords account, you have the ability to start a radio advertising campaign right from your computer. It is a great tool to use!

Newspapers - local newspaper or magazine ads can be placed from your adwords account as well.

Community flyer postings- spas, MD offices, gyms, grocery stores, pharmacies, hospital lobbies are great places to display your flyers.

Personal Selling

Even with all the marketing efforts above, you still come to a point where you have to make contact with a potential client and make them aware of the benefits of your service and why your service is a perfect match for their needs. Here are some powerful questions that allow the potential client to sell themselves on your program:

"What is it about coaching that sounds most interesting?"

"How do you think you would benefit from partnering with a coach?"

"What would be different if you worked with a coach?"

"Is there something you would like some help with right now?"

"How ready are you to reach your goals?"

"What is motivating you at this point in your life?

"If you did hire a coach, where would you like to start your coaching work?"

"How much would it be worth to you to solve your problems?"

"Have you ever considered having a coach of your own?"

"What can't you do for yourself that perhaps a partner like a coach could help you do?"

"What questions do you have about coaching?"

"May I tell you a little bit about a client I have worked with, who was facing something similar?"

We are continually developing new ways for you to market and sell your service as an RN Health Coach. We offer a variety of marketing pieces such as brochures and letters, and they are always changing. The pieces would incorporate a branded image, logo and a clear and concise message about the service, the expertise and the benefits of the business.

Business cards are provided as part of your start-up kit. You may order more by contacting us.

Price, Product, Placement or Distribution and Position or Market share are all classic marketing elements. Setting the price and defining the product are critical elements. They should be done in view of the competition and the emerging trends in the field as well as the limiting factors of what you have determined you are looking for in terms of new income.

Market share and distribution are often determined by the use of a mixed media approach which could include: print ads, newspaper or magazine ads, TV commercials, radio ads, and press releases.

The cost for traditional marketing can be significant. It is essential to know your business well and to be clear, concise and consistent in the branding of the business.

Internet Marketing Strategies

The rise in the power of search engines and internet usage has opened new doors for promotion and branding.

For most businesses this begins with the website. The website should echo the image you have for

49

your business. We provide you with a URL that you can direct potential clients to. The format of the URL is www.RNHealthCoach.com/FirstName/. You have the ability via your admin section to update and customize your profile. If you would like to purchase your own URL, such as www.yourname.com we can assist you in that and point the new domain name to your profile page.

Articles, eBooks and blogs will generate more search engine visibility as well as enhancing the expertise concept for your brand.

Other Internet Marketing Strategies may include:

- Entering information in Industry Specific Directories.
- Arrange for cross links to other sites.
- Consider web affiliation or web rings.
- Apply for industry specific awards.
- Post on newsgroups, blogs, wikis and forums.
- Offer a membership with cross linking.
- List the site in professional association directories.
- Share knowledge through articles, eBooks, Books and lists.
- Offer related resources.
- Use eNewsletters or eTip broadcasts to build business.
- Use press releases to drive up web traffic.
- Consider adwords or other SEO program to build Search Engine Optimization (SEO).
- Offer Teleclasses.
- Host discussion groups.
- Run contests.

Partnerships, Referrals and Relationship Channels

Consider partnering with physicians, therapists and other professionals for cross referrals. Also consider asking for permission to leave brochures or flyers in waiting rooms. Make sure you can answer questions other professionals might have, and stress the fact that you want to work together.

Your service can be a strong asset for a medical practice that sees overweight and obese clients. They may not have the time or personnel to spend the time necessary to support the weight loss and wellness strategies that your business will be centered on.

Contact local companies, especially those that employ large numbers of employees to see if you can create a discounted program or special offer for their company.

In many cases, employers have seen the benefit of health coaching in reducing absenteeism and improving productivity as well as increasing employee loyalty. These employers may be interested in paying for or off-setting the cost of your services.

Press and Article Ideas

Press releases can be distributed electronically through press wire services, or you can build your own list of media contacts and develop a press kit to support your business brand. The press kit should include a business card, brochure, articles, both published and unpublished, previous press releases and other information about your business, credentials and services. Consider some of the following ideas for press release, eBooks and articles:

- Baby Boomers and RN Health Coaches
- Improving Employee Performance with RN Health Coaches
- Tele-Coaching: Taking the Pain from the Process
- RN Health Coaching: Simplify the Process

51

Unfinished Business

Business structure

Some thought should be given to how you would like to structure your business. Generally, your choices are sole proprietor, partnership or corporation. You can view a comparison of these at the following sites, as well as set up:

Legalzoom.com – Recommended

Bizfilings.com

Incorporate.com

Dress code

It is recommended you wear a scrub top or lab coat during your interactions with clients. The top should have your credentials and business logo (you may use ours, of course). Wearing such "medical" attire reinforces your position as a medical professional, which is what differentiates our service and also allows you to brand your business and name as a coach.

Insurance

You may find it a good idea to get some professional liability insurance to cover your practice as a nurse educator and RN Health Coach. Check out www.nso.com to obtain your professional liability insurance and protect yourself and business from any risk.

Where to Get Free Counseling

- Small Business Development Centers www.sba.gov/gopher/local-information/small-business-development-centers/
- SCORE www.score.org
- Chambers of Commerce http://chamber-of-commerce.com/

Sources of Start-Up Funds

- microLoan programs 800-827-5722
- www.venturea.com

Where to Find Grants

- www.cfda.gov
- www.cof.org

Selling to the government

- www.bidservices.com
- cbdnet.access.gpo.gov
- www.merxbidline.com

Client Educational Literature

- www.channing-bete.com

52

L.I.T.E. Behaviors: Owning Success

The objective in Health Coaching is to build buy-in from the client. This is their responsibility and the work and effort will be theirs to embrace.

The urge may be to jump in with both feet and facilitate the process strongly. But it is important that the RN Health Coach is not doing more work than the client in the effort to redirect his or her lifestyle. If they do not own the process, they cannot own the success.

In your "clients" section of the website, there is an area entitled L.I.T.E. Behaviors and Goals. Have your clients look at this section and pick from the list of behaviors and/or goals to work on until the next time you meet. At this time you will review the goal and hold the client accountable for it as well as set up a new goal for the following meeting. This is the magic of our program and why it works!

Measure and Monitor

Consider how you will track progress. Will you look at measurement, weight and circumference numbers or will you want to include a broader spectrum of metrics? These may include cholesterol, glucose and other blood indicators of wellness and health.

Will you monitor flexibility, fitness and stress test levels? Will you track lung capacity and endurance levels? Will you keep markers for emotional milestones?

Will you create a reward and recognition system to keep the client aware of progress and enhance the motivation process?

Goal Setting and Goal Attainment

It is critical to your success that the goals are clear, concise and agreed upon by both the RN Health Coach and the client.

Track progress and keep the feedback immediate and direct.

53

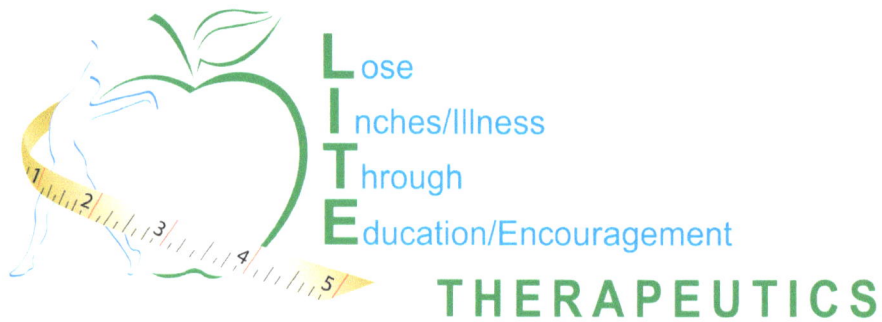

For Free Training On How To Become A RN Health Coach Visit:

www.HealthCoachNursingJobs.com

Weight Loss Coaching

There are many different approaches to weight loss. The healthiest way to lose weight is to reduce the amount of calories you consume and to increase your level of activity, simple as that. After reading this section you will have an understanding of how to help your client achieve their weight loss goals by changing and keeping track of the foods they eat. You will have an understanding of how the body utilizes the calories we consume and how the sources of calories we ingest make a difference in weight loss.

Some clients choose to use medication or over the counter supplements to aid in weight loss. We have tried to cover some of these aids in this chapter. Keep in mind that new medications and aids are engineered everyday and not all are healthy for your client. Familiarize yourself with "alternative or non-traditional" weight loss medications and supplements so that you are not caught off guard when asked about this topic. ALWAYS insist that before your client decide to take any medication whether OTC or prescribed, your client has thoroughly discussed it with their primary medical doctor.

Nutrients

Not all calories are created equal. Food should be viewed as a drug. To shift your paradigm toward this belief can be the most powerful thing you can do for your health. Foods, like drugs, have a specific effect, specific interactions and specific side effects. There is a metabolic, hormonal and chemical response that follows their intake.

There are no such things as bad food, only bad choices and bad timing

Let's look into some nutrient sources, such as fats, carbs (carbohydrates) and proteins:

Fats

Fats yield the highest calories per gram when compared to carbs or protein. Fats yield 9 calories per gram vs. 4 from the other two. Gram for gram, they produce more energy than the other two. We also expend very little fuel in digesting fats. We access 97-100% of the calories from fat.

Fats also do not take up much space in the stomach compared to the other two, so we may tend to eat it more of them.

Fat is very good at providing the feeling of fullness.

55

When meal planning, limit your fat to no more than 20% (30% max) of your total caloric intake. Let's do the math:

1,200 cal daily diet

1,200 x .20 = 240 calories

In this example, don't consume more than 240 cal (calories) of fat for the day. Since it is easier to count in terms of grams of fat for the day, let's convert.

9 cal of fat = 1 gm, so:

240 cal / 9 = 26.6 or 27 grams of fat limit for the day.

It is much easier to count the grams of fat on food labels rather than totaling calories, so count in terms of grams.

To help aid in the reduction of fat intake, one may consider a drug that inhibits the lipase enzyme and blocks fat absorption by 30%. This can be prescribed or purchased over the counter as Alli. Encourage your client to research or look into this if fats represent a large portion of their diet. Make sure they ask their doctor if this would be of some help.

Carbohydrates

Carbohydrates are derived from non-animal foods. They are foods that are grown.

Carbs are a primary and essential source of energy.

All carbs are broken down and absorbed as sugar or blood glucose.

The amount of time involved in this breakdown or absorption is fast or slow. High-glycemic index carbs are broken down very quickly and trigger a fast release of insulin. Low-glycemic carbs have a slower breakdown of sugar and thus a slower and steadier release of insulin.

Different types of carbs will have either a high or low effect on the hormonal and biochemical systems of the body. They will cause either a high rise in blood sugar and insulin or a low rise with minimal or no rise in serum insulin levels. The body constantly monitors the amount of sugar in the blood. It likes this range to be between 70-110mg. As sugar/glucose levels rise toward or above 110 the body will release a clearing or storage hormone called insulin to take the excess sugar out the blood and store it in the muscle, liver or fat tissue. On the other end, when sugar levels approach or fall below 70, the body releases a "liberating" or breakdown hormone called glucagon to pull sugar out of muscle, the liver or even fatty acid to drag it back into the blood.

At any given time you are either liberating or storing fat.

Let's look at the muscle and liver which store sugar as glycogen as if they were a cup. The cup can only hold so much sugar. When the cup is only half full (or half empty) your body will utilize energy from carbohydrates AND fat. Now as the cup becomes more full the body will utilize energy from carbs and leave fat alone. When your cup is full and you consume too much carbs, your cup will "run over" and the excess is stored as fat. On the opposite end, when your cup is empty, the body turns toward fat for energy.

56

Glycemic Index GI

GI is the rate blood glucose levels rise after eating foods, with 0 being the lowest or no rise, and 100 being the fastest rise. Buy yourself a book listing levels of glycemic index for food items. Have your clients eat low on this list or reserve the high items for only the first couple of hours in the morning, when they have the majority of the day to burn them off.

The more refined, processed or cooked the carb is, the faster it breaks down into glucose which in turn, affects insulin levels. Manufactured carbs cause the release, calorie for calorie, of more insulin than natural carbs.

200 calories of yams will cause less insulin release than 200 calories of pretzels or potato chips.

Insulin

Insulin is responsible for getting sugar out of the blood and into tissues such as muscles and fat. The amount of insulin released is related to the concentration of glucose in the blood, and the concentration is related to your total carbohydrate intake.

Your goal should be to lower the need for excessive insulin in the blood.

For every item you put in your mouth, you should think, how will this affect my insulin levels?

High insulin levels are a result of eating above your caloric requirements or from eating fast-digesting carbs within your caloric requirements that promote fat storage. This often results from a highly refined diet with almost no fiber and lots of simple sugars. Elevated insulin levels keep the body from tapping into body fat stores.

High levels of insulin are also an appetite stimulant.

High insulin levels release an enzyme called lipoprotein lipase (LPL). This enzyme retards the fat cells and prevents them from being broken apart to be used up as fuel.

Glucagon

The effects of glucagon are the opposite of insulin.

It promotes the release of HSL (hormone sensitive lipase) which works on fat cells to liberate fatty acids. It puts them into the blood where they can be used.

Adding glucagon to insulin lowers the insulin level and its fat-storing ability. This can be done by consuming protein with carbohydrate meals.

For meal planning, carbs can range from 5%-50% of caloric intake.

Ketogenic diets: 5%-15%

Low carb diet: 25%-30%

Moderate: 40-50%

Fiber

Fiber is a non-digestible food substance.

The body expends more energy to break down fiber than it gets from its absorption.

Fiber also slows the rate of absorption of carbs. This means less of an insulin spike and less glucose release.

As a coach you should encourage the use of fiber when appropriate. Encourage clients to use an odorless and tasteless fiber supplement to slow the absorption of higher glycemic index carbs.

It is possible to stay within your caloric limits and create an environment where insulin levels remain chronically high making it almost impossible to lose fat. This occurs when there is low fiber or when one consumes high glycemic-index foods producing insulin spikes.

Consume at least 25-30 grams of fiber per day

Sugars

Total sugar consumption should be limited 6% of total caloric intake.

For example, if you are on a 2,000 cal diet, 6% = .06 x 2,000= 120 cal.

120 cal. divided by 4 (the number of cal. per gram) = 30gm. No more than 30 gms of sugar per day should be consumed! Stick to this and the pounds will melt away! Start counting the grams of sugar.

Alpha-glucosidase enzyme inhibitor

This is an enzyme involved in breaking down simple carbohydrates. Certain agents can decrease the breakdown of simple carbs resulting in a slower and lower rise in blood glucose.

Acarbose (RX drug) 50mg three times a day

Alpha-amylase inhibitor

These agents interfere with the breakdown of large carbohydrate molecules.

White kidney bean extract (OTC supplement)

Protein

Protein comes from animal products. All proteins are broken down into amino acids.

Protein has the highest thermic effect of the macronutrient food groups. It takes more energy or calories to digest proteins than it does fats or carbohydrates. 20-30% of calories in protein are lost as heat in the digestion process. (You can eat more for less.)

Proteins cause the release of insulin and glucagon, with glucagon being the greater of the two released.

For meal planning, protein should range from 10%-35% of caloric intake.

Water

To determine the amount of water needed in a day, take your scale weight in pounds and multiple it by 0.75. This will give you the amount of fluid in ounces.

See your resource CD that came with your kit for an Excel program that can calculate nutrient ratios of fat, protein and carbs.

Food timing

Generally, the body will not utilize fat when sugar is present to burn and use for energy.

Our bodies are designed to do this for survival. We try to protect the fat for an upcoming starvation period. If we repeatedly consume high glycemic carbs all day, spiking our insulin levels, we set up an environment for fat storage, which is what our bodies are designed to do. The body may use its current carbs and is not required to turn to fat for energy until a period of starvation.

We must trick the body!

We do this by decreasing the amount of sugar/carbs, thereby decreasing the insulin and forcing the body to turn to fat stores.

Make your body burn fat by decreasing the high glycemic carbs as well as total calories throughout the day.

Insulin the wrong way!

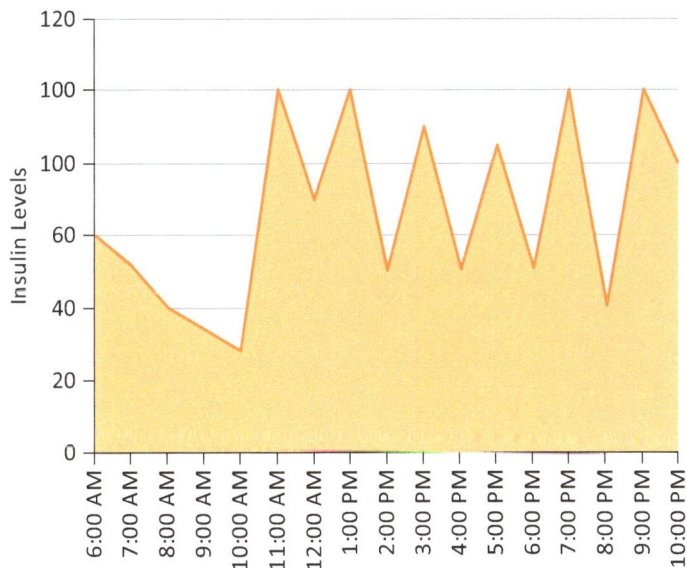

59

Insulin the right way!

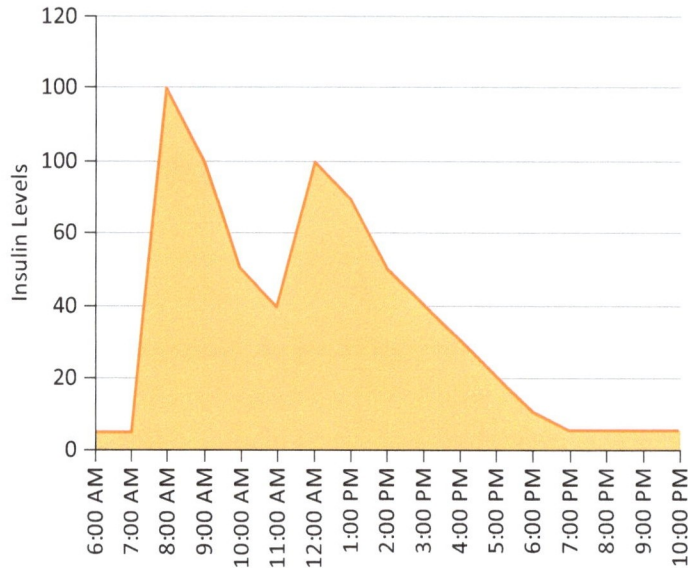

When you time the foods you eat with other daily events, you optimize the intake of that food. Better yet, you optimize the affect the food has on you.

Taper your carbs throughout the day. Try this - The *only* carbs you should consume after 2:30 pm (for us normal-day folks) must be either salad or vegetables, no fruit, no other source of carbs! No kidding! Following this regimen will have you burning fat like fire! You will have switched your metabolism to one that burns fat for energy rather than carbs.

Defining fat

Measuring fat distribution helps to calculate the risk of co-morbidities that exist with obesity. Below are some objective measures of obesity:

BMI

BMI is a ratio of weight to height. It is the same for both sexes. BMI Charts can be found online and many other places. Risks associated with an increased BMI begin at >25.

Here are the classifications:

<18 - underweight

18.5-24.9 - normal range

25-29.9 – overweight: "increased" risk of co-morbidity

30-34.9 - class I obesity: "Moderate" risk of co-morbidity

35-39.9 - class II obesity: "Severe" risk of co-morbidity

>40 - class III obesity: "Very Severe" risk of co-morbidity

60

There are some limitations with using BMI. It does not account for proportion of fat versus lean body mass, or the location of excess fat. An athlete with increased muscle mass may have a BMI >30 but little fat. An older person who has lost a lot of muscle mass, may have a BMI <25 but carry excess fat in the abdominal area.

Waist circumference

Waist circumference is measured at the midpoint between the lower border of the rib cage and iliac crest. Obesity by this measure is defined as:

Men >40 inches

Women > 35 inches

Abdominal fat is strongly associated with type 2 diabetes and other metabolic risks.

Waist to hip ratio

To obtain this ratio, measure the waist circumference and divide by the hip circumference.

Obesity is then defined as:

Men >1.0

Women > 0.85

Body fat percentage

This measurement is obtained by dividing the amount of weight in fat by total body weight

Description	Women	Men
Essential fat	10–12%	2–4%
Athletes	14–20%	6–13%
Fitness	21–24%	14–17%
Acceptable	25–31%	18–25%
Overweight	32-41%	26-37%
Obese	42%+	38%+

It is suggested you record all of the above measurements when you follow up with your clients.

Why diets don t work

1. Too much serum insulin in the blood caused by Insulin resistance.

When muscle receptors are dull and the pancreas reacts by kicking insulin levels into overdrive, carbs are diverted away from glycogen stores (your cups) and stored as body fat.

Resistance muscle 1}leads to more insulin release and encourages fat storage.

Building muscle can increase your ability to store glycogen and improve your ability to draw glucose out of the blood and into the muscle instead of fat cells.

61

Agents that may increase insulin sensitivity

1. Fiber

2. Omega-3's

3. Chromium supplement

Items that increase insulin resistance
Stress
Smoking
Lack of exercise
Alcohol
Low fiber diet
High sugar diet
Recreational drugs
High amount of body fat

2. **Diet-Induced Reduction of Metabolic rate**

Reduction in caloric intake causes a decrease in T3 (thyroid hormone) levels. The lowering of T3 lowers the basal metabolic rate and favors conservation of energy.

3. **Depletion of lean tissue**

The way we often diet, with huge caloric deficits, causes muscle mass to be lost at ratio of 1:1 muscle and fat. With the loss of muscle we also decrease our metabolic rate.

Assessing caloric need

The amount of calories one consumes should never be below one's BMR (basal metabolic rate). This is the number of calories required daily to maintain muscle mass and to provide fuel for the organs and brain. It is the bare minimum required to maintain life. Eating a diet below one's BMR will burn protein from muscles and organs, leading to less muscle and a lower metabolism as the body will adjust itself to make it through each day on fewer total calories.

After finding one's BMR, we must provide additional fuel to perform daily work and exercise. The amount added is based on activity and lifestyle.

Non-active = no exercise or works a non-physical job.

$$BMR \times 0.2 + BMR$$

Moderately Active= desk job and works out 3-4 times a week or a physical job and does not exercise.

$$BMR \times 0.4 + BMR$$

Very Active = either works a physical job and exercises 3 times a week or works a desk job and works out hard 5 times a week.

$$BMR \times 0.7 + BMR$$

62

Extremely Active= works a physical job, construction, mail carrier, builder and works out hard 5 or more times each week.

$$BMR \times 1 + BMR$$

So to calculate an example, the caloric need for an active individual with a moderately-active lifestyle with a BMR of 1,200, we will do the following math:

$(1,200 \times 0.4)= 480 +1,200= 1,680$

So 1,680 would be the amount needed to maintain their weight.

How do we calculate BMR?

BMR can be calculated in many ways. The most respected and accurate is the Harris-Benedict equation. You can search online for the formula if you wish to use it.

We will use another formula which we find easier to use. It is as follows:

Male: *LEAN Mass* in lbs x 12.5=BMR

Or

Scale weight in lbs x 11 =BMR

Women: *LEAN mass* in lbs x 11=BMR

Or

Scale weight in lbs x 10 =BMR

Now that you know to calculate BMR, don't forget to add the activity component to come up with the **total** calories needed.

Here are some caloric needs assessment calculators found online:

www.bodybuilding.com/fun/par8.htm

www.bodybuilding.com/fun/issa64.htm

www.bodybuilding.com/fun/calrmr.htm

www.bodybuilding.com/fun/calcal.htm

Creating proper caloric deficit
Coax fat loss, don't force it.

Reduce your determined caloric intake as we calculated above by only 15%-20%. For example if it takes 2,000 cal a day to maintain your current weight and we aim for a 15% reduction, then 2,000 x 0.15= 300, so reduce your calories by 300 per day which would now equal 2,000-300= 1,700

Never fall below your BMR.
The trick is to stimulate and encourage the body to liberate fat without setting off an alarm in the fat cells, where they fight back and resist being broken down, and T3 levels decline.

There is tons of meal planning software out there. This may be an excellent tool to add to your service.

63

Getting to know the hormones involved in weight loss

There are several hormones that impact how many calories are stored as fat. If any of these hormones are out of balance, one can gain weight even if while eating less food. Let's take a look at 5 of these hormones. As an RN Health Coach your role is to identify any one of these hormones as a possible contributor to weight-loss prevention and bring this to the attention of the client so they may seek a remedy from their doctor. Remember you only identify and inform. It is their doctor that diagnoses and treats. Later I will explain how you can coordinate these lab studies and charge for this, adding an additional revenue stream to your income.

You do need to know that not all physicians agree about some of the following information. The handling of thyroid hormone replacement and the use of certain drugs may vary considerably from one doctor to the next. If either you or your client is insistent on a specific medication you want the doctor to prescribe, or a test you want him to order, be aware that not every doctor will agree with you. You may find doctors who suggest that what you want to do could be very unsafe. You can find the phone number to reach doctors that agree with much of this information a little further on in this handbook.

In reviewing lab results, it is important to distinguish "normal" levels from "optimal" levels

1. Insulin

Insulin has a significant effect on both hunger and fat storage. The net effect of insulin is the storage of carbohydrate, protein and fat in the body. Even in caloric restriction or dieting excess, insulin prevents stored body fat from being released. It is possible for blood glucose levels to be normal, yet serum insulin levels to be beyond normal range. Not only does high serum insulin or hyperinsulinemia prevent fat loss but it appears to promote hypertension by impairing sodium balance, and causes harm to the kidneys and vascular system. It also may increase the risk and progression of certain cancers by acting as a catalyst to cell growth.

Laboratory reference ranges indicate "normal" levels of fasting insulin as 6-27 mclU/ml. These levels in the obese often exceed 20. For **optimal health, this level should be in the range of 0-3**.

Those clients that are prescribed metformin (brand name Glucophage) should be encouraged to stay in compliance with this medicine. It can promote insulin sensitivity to the cells and also inhibit some carbohydrate absorption. The net effect is a lesser need of insulin secretion as a better job is obtained moving glucose to the cells with less production.

Don't forget about Alpha-glucosidase enzyme inhibitors and Alpha-amylase inhibitors mentioned in the carb section.

For chronically high levels of fasting insulin you may need to stop eating after 6:30 pm and/or consume only low glycemic-index foods.

2. Thyroid

Some physicians believe that most people over 40 have a subclinical thyroid deficiency that contributes to their weight gain (Bemben et al. 1994; Samuels 1998).

64

A hypoactive thyroid can result in the slowing down of the body's metabolic rate.

Clients with thyroid deficiency should be prescribed drugs such as Cytomel or Armour 1}under the supervision of a doctor. Many people become thyroid deficient in response to dieting. Also drugs like metformin or appetite suppressants may make one thyroid deficient because of the reduced intake of calories. If T3 levels are not in the upper one third range of normal, consider asking MD for replacement therapy.

T3 measurement can determine how much metabolically active thyroid hormone is available to the tissues. The normal T3 range is 2.3-4.2 pg/ml but for losing weight, you might want the range to be between 3.4-4.2. If the range is below this, advocate for treating with Cytomel 12.5mcg twice daily.

If T3 levels are above normal, this can indicate an overdose of drugs or hyperthyroidism.

If TSH levels are high, this means that the pituitary gland is over-secreting a hormone to stimulate thyroid function because of a deficiency. Remember, there is an inverse relationship between TSH and thyroid function. The higher the TSH level, the more likely the client is to be thyroid deficient. The normal TSH range can be as wide as 0.2-5.5 mIU/ml. However if TSH levels are above 2.0, consider a benefit from the drug Cytomel or Armour.

T4 Normal range of T4 is 4.5-12mcg/dl. **For weight loss aim for the upper half of this range, above 8.5**.

If there is too much T4, this is a sign of hyperthyroidism that should receive immediate medical treatment.

3. Estradiol and Progesterone

Estradiol

Men: goal range 10-30 pg/ml

If estradiol levels are high in men over 30, asking a MD for **Arimidex** 0.5mg twice a week to block the conversion of testosterone to estrogen may provide some benefit.

Obese Postmenopausal women range in 50-150pg/ml

The goal should be the lowest amount needed to be symptom-free. Postmenopausal women who are not taking estrogen drugs are normally around 30pg/ml.

Women deficient in estrogen are predisposed to abdominal fat accumulation. Women with levels below 90pg/ml could benefit from a prescribed compounded bioidentical estriol/estradiol cream to increase levels above 90.

Women with existing estrogen-receptor positive cancers should not take estrogen.

Progesterone
Postmenopausal women. Goal >2.0ng/ml

Balancing estradiol levels in women is complicated and individualistic. The general relation of progesterone to estradiol in healthy women is around 10:1.

65

Referrals to MD's knowledgeable in hormonal regulation can be found at 800-226-2370.

Because of the complexity of women's hormone replacement, visit www.lef.org/estrogen for more information.

Again, this is an area of controversy. If a client's doctor does not agree, and the client likes his or her doctor and gets good medical care, you and the client should think carefully about damaging that relationship if the doctor does not agree with this type of hormone manipulation.

4. Testosterone

Healthy testosterone levels are necessary for both men and women. Be careful of eating high fat foods; this may reduce free testosterone levels, according to one study. The drug metformin can also have the side effect of lowering testosterone.

Free testosterone

Men

Quest lab: 150-200 pg/ml

LabCorp: 18-26

Men should have a PSA test also to rule out prostate cancer.

If free testosterone is below optimal range, recommend asking a physician for a prescription for trans-dermal cream providing 5 mg a day.

Women 1.0-2.5 pg/ml

5. DHEA

The adrenal hormone dehydroepiandrosterone or DHEA has been associated with many benefits. The levels of DHEA are high in our youth, and then start to decline as we age. The theory is that we can guard against age-related health issues; the goal with DHEA is to replace to levels of youthfulness. **DHEA is contraindicated in men and women with hormone-related cancers**. Men should have a PSA done before they begin replacement therapy. The average daily dose for men is 50 mg and 15-50 mg daily for women. This can be purchased over the counter. Have your clients test their levels for a baseline, then again after some weeks of treatment.

Men: goal range 400-560mcg/dl

Women: goal range 350-430mcg/dl

In summary:

- **If fasting insulin is high, it could be suppressed.**
- **If thyroid is low, there may be benefit to bring back to normal.**
- **Estrogen, testosterone, and DHEA could be restored to youthful levels based on your assessment and PMD cooperation/approval.**

Approaching the PMD

If a patient shows up in a doctor's office with a list of things a Health Coach wants done, the response of the doctor may not be what you would want. A much better approach would be, I have this information. Is there anything in this that you think might help me? For example, could my thyroid be low? Most doctors are reasonable, but don't want to be told what to do.

Having labs drawn

The labs that we identified above can be requested from the client's physician. They can have their PMD draw these labs. However, if there is an issue with their doctors drawing the labs, or insurance reimbursement issues, you can coordinate the drawing of these labs for a fee. This may offer convenience for your client as well as a source of income for you. Your fees can be edited from the admin section of your site.

How do you coordinate lab draws?

It is easy. Join this organization: www.lef.org (Life Extension). It is a great organization to belong to. You will keep up to date on the latest progressive research. As a member, you can order labs on the behalf of someone else for a discounted fee. Use this organization to set up a lab draw, give them the name of the individual you are purchasing this gift for, and have your client show up for the draw. It's as easy as that.

Remember to tell your clients not to eat 12 hours prior to labs being drawn.

Also, another lab not mentioned above is C - reactive protein. You may have heard of it regarding heart disease. This is a marker of chronic inflammation. It contributes to obesity by binding to the hormone leptin. Leptin helps signal satiety, thereby reducing hunger, and promotes the breakdown of lipolysis. It may be a good idea to offer this lab also.

Medications

Your client should be made aware of all possible options available to them. There are several FDA-approved drugs available to treat obesity. The following site can be viewed for more information. You can even print a PDF version of the publication to hand to clients as a guide. They will appreciate you for this. Here is the site: http://win.niddk.nih.gov/publications/prescription.htm

Treatment with meds usually must meet the following criteria:

BMI >30

BMI >27 with 2 or more obesity-related complications.

Here are some RX drugs:

Phentermine - appetite suppressant. Use as short-term management, up to 12 weeks.

Xenical - lipase inhibitor. Blocks up to 30% of fat intake. Available over the counter in half-dose form as **Alli. Be sure to discuss the side effects of this drug with your clients and encourage client communication with PMD regarding any medications.**

67

Meridia

Metformin

Any client presenting with any indications of metabolic syndrome, prediabetes, or type 2 diabetes should be made aware of possible benefit from this drug. It can help suppress appetite while improving the metabolic profile. Any client with symptoms of **diabetes who has not been diagnosed needs to see a physician.**

Screen for meds that may cause weight gain

Screen for any possible medication that may cause weight gain and have the client along with their physician evaluate the need to continue with it. This is a discussion they should have with their physician.

- Glucocorticoids
- Tricyclic and heterocyclic antidepressants
- Lithium
- Phenothiazides
- Sulphonylurea agents
- Estrogens
- Cyproheptadine

Supplements

Go over possible dietary supplements that may help. Here are a few.

CLA

CLA is a fatty acid that may reduce body fat, aid in muscle development and energy production. This supplement has been shown to decrease the volume of adipocytes by reducing the capacity of them to store fat.

In studies, results were achieved with 3-4 grams a day.

Omega -3 s

These essential fatty acids can aid in weight loss by promoting thermogenesis, in which foods are converted to heat, and also by making cell membranes more sensitive to the effects of insulin - leading to less production of the hormone for its effects.

Chromium

Use to improve insulin sensitivity.
200 mcg with each meal

Magnesium

Magnesium has an important role in carbohydrate metabolism. A deficiency in this may cause insulin resistance. Many people are deficient. You can test for this electrolyte in a chemistry panel to make sure. For those going on a calorie restricted diet, a dose of 300-500 mg can be taken a day.

Fiber

Fiber can increase post-meal satiety, or sensation of fullness, and decrease subsequent hunger. Fiber also slows the absorption of carbs to make for a more even release of insulin instead of quick, rapid, insulin spikes.

Take at least 25-30 grams a day. Do not consume with fatty acid supplements.

White kidney bean extract

Researchers have found an extract in white kidney beans may help the body stop carbs from breaking down into sugars.

Below are the 4 components of our program:

1. **Assessment**

Vitals
Body fat, waist circumference, hip to waist
Screening Cholesterol, Blood Glucose
Caloric intake
Hormonal
Dietary supplements, meds

2. **L.I.T.E. Diet**
   1. **Caloric reduction**

      A) Counting grams method. Determine the ratio of protein, fats and carbs. Convert them into grams. Keep a daily running tally of allotted grams of fat, proteins, carbs and sugar.

      B) Plate method. If you feel your client cannot be compliant with the counting method, as it does require effort, then a simple, easy method of restricting calories and creating a a caloric deceit may be the plate method. Here is how it works. Divide a plate in half, now half of that plate can be dedicated to fruits and vegetables. Now the next step, divide the other half of the plate into half, so you have1/4 and 1/4 of the original. In one component, place your meats, and the other can be a starch or carb. This plate method is a way to prevent overeating.

      Check out www.portiondoctor.com to order your own branded portion control plates.
   2. **Protein and fiber with every meal.**
   3. **Eat every 3 hours.**
   4. **No carbs, except salad and vegetables after 2:30.**
   5. **Calorie free drinks.**

69

3. L.I.T.E. Exercise

Research as pointed out a "magic" number of 10,000 steps per day as the amount of activity needed to classify one as "active." We at L.I.T.E. Therapeutics support this method of exercise and activity. The 10,000 step program requires your client to use a pedometer to account for the amount of activity via movement/walking they perform in a day. Most people will walk about 900-3,000 steps per day. So it is clear that some "extra" activity or walking is required to reach the 10,000 goal.

Here is a breakdown of activity levels classifications depending on steps walked per day:

Under 5,000 = sedentary lifestyle

5,000-7,499 = low active

7,500- 9,999 = somewhat active

10,000 = active

12,500+ = highly active

Once your client gets a baseline of the steps they walk per day, they should aim at a goal of 500 more steps per week.

Walking the equivalent of 10,000 steps is close to 5 miles and walking this will burn 300-500 calories.

Walking throughout the day with a pedometer is a fun and easy way to stay active. You can also provide branded pedometers to your client from the marketing section of your site to ensure you stay on your clients mind!

Here are some other fitness guidelines:

- Never perform more than 90 minutes of continuous intense cardio. After this point you will be burning muscle and killing your metabolism.
- Workout at an intensity of 55-80% of your maximum heart rate. Max heart rate is 220-your age. For example, for a 30 year old: 220-30=190 maximum heart rate. 60% of this .60x 190=114.
- The best time to perform cardio is first thing in the morning on an empty stomach. The amount of glucose in the blood influences how fast the body will dig into fat stores.

4. L.I.T.E. Motivation

See chapter on motivational interviewing.

Below is a sample 16 week weight loss coaching schedule. The beginning of every month provides a personal visit and assessment followed by weekly phone follow ups and support group meetings (outsourced).

Example 16 week session
Week 1
Assessment, measurements, screening, labs, diet.
On the first visit, you will meet personally with the client. Ensure you are dressed appropriately with lab coat or scrub top. Give the image of a healthcare professional. Prior to the visit you should

70

complete the American Heart BP and diabetes risk calculator located in the assessment section of our clients' management area in your admin section of the site.

When you see the clients, present the data from the risk calculator.

Perform a physical assessment, consisting of:

- Blood glucose screening.

- Cholesterol point of care screening.

- Vital signs. BP, HR, Respiratory rate, etc.

- Body fat measurements, scale weight.

- Review of any previous lab results.

During this encounter give a brief overview of your program. Explain basic elements of nutrients and the L.I.T.E. Diet.

Have the client set a goal for the following week telephone follow-up call.

Arrange a time and date for the phone follow up.

Send an email reminder.

Week 2-4 (follow up)
TOPS, weekly phone f/u, weigh-ins, goal setting & review.

Optional - During the week, have your client attend a TOPS support group (www.tops.org). This is a very inexpensive program. You can sponsor your client's session. You can factor this cost in when you price your program, but the cost is very minimal. You can also brand your service as a coach at the local chapter.

Call client for your phone appointment.

Let client know you have x minutes allotted for this phone follow up (very important).

Discuss success of goal that was set week prior.

Obtain weight for the week.

Theme for remaining weeks is diet, so you may inform about any aspect of diet and nutrition.

Have client set goal for next week. Remember goals are set on clients' website.

Obtain time for next personal meeting.

Week 5
Assessment, measurements, Fitness theme

Same as week one meeting, except goal and discussions are fitness related.

Obtain measurements, goals.

Obtain time and date for next follow up.

Week 6-8 (follow up)

TOPS meetings, weekly phone f/u, weigh in, goal setting & review.

Same weekly follow up format from week 2-4.

Fitness-related goals and discussion in addition to diet goals.

Hold accountable for previous goals.

Give or leave info on fitness topics.

Week 9

Assessment, measurements, Disease/Condition, Health Optimization

Personal visit.

Same as week one, but with disease and condition information specific to them, to guide conversation. In addition to diet and fitness, they now add goals relating to their condition.

Week 10-13 (follow up)

Follow up visit template. Same as above.

Goals now include condition-specific or disease-prevention topics.

Obtain scale weight.

Hold accountable for last week's goals, set new goals.

Give or leave information regarding topic.

Week 14 Personal visit/Motivation theme.

Week 15-16 (follow up)
Your goals as a L.I.T.E. Weight Loss Coach:

- Restore insulin sensitivity.
- Restore youthful hormone balance.
- Control rate of carbohydrate absorption.
- Increase physical activity.
- Restore /maintain resting energy expenditure rate.
- Aim for a 0.5-2 lb weight loss per week.

Anything greater, you are likely burning protein or muscle which will lower your BMR.
- Keeping insulin levels low, avoiding excess fat and avoiding excess calories are key!
- Put your body in a position metabolically where you are not storing any additional fat, then work off your existing fat by increasing your metabolic rate via exercise, eating often(every 3 hours), eating proteins and fiber.

Smoking Cessation Coaching

Coaching services in attempts to help others quit smoking can be provided as a stand-alone service, or in conjunction with your weight loss coaching, as a added bonus to help stimulate sales at a discounted rate, or even free. The amount of face-to-face contact should be at least 90 minutes minimum. One 90 minute session is not advised. Sessions should be divided up, to anywhere between 4-8 sessions lasting greater than 10 minutes each. It is common to front-load sessions so that several occur during the first week or two of quiting when risk of lapse is high. Face-to-face contact can be augmented by phone or email, which is not counted toward the 90 minutes. It is recommended that you as a coach charge for your time. Determine the length of time for your program and charge accordingly. If your program is 2 hours in length and your rate is $100/hour, then your smoking cessation program would be $200.

Why Coaching For Smoking Cessation?

-Quitting Success is Low without Counseling/Coaching
-Coaching Addresses Obstacles to Quitting That Medications Cannot
-Coaching Can Enhance Medication Effects

Fewer than 3% of smokers who try to quit independently succeed(CDCP, 3005a).

Quiting smoking is about breaking strong associations with environmental stimuli, such as cues or triggers associated with nicotine use. It is not likely that medications alone with solve this. Also the uses of meds are limited. For these reasons a Health Coach such as you is needed.

Getting a client to quit smoking is the most important behavior change of all!

To deliver effective coaching to help quit smoking, one must have a good understanding of the health consequences of tobacco dependence. This information will help enhance your clients' motivation to quit.

- Smoking tobacco kills 5 million people wordwide(Ezzati & Lopez, 2003), or about one person every 6 seconds.

- It shortens good quality of life 1}by an average of 10 years (Doll, Peto, Boreham, & Sutherland, 2004).

- Smoking increases the risk of death due to lung cancer by more than 10 times (US Department of Helath and Human Services, 1989).

- Smoking more than doubles the risk for myocardial infarction and related heart disease.

73

- Women who smoke have a more difficult time becoming pregnant, have a greater risk of spontaneous abortion, and give birth to babies lower in weight and more likely to die from SIDS.

- Smoking is associated with reduced sexual function in men.

- Smoking increases facial wrinkles.

You will never be short of clients in this area. Nearly 50 million Americans smoke and 1 billion worldwide. Help from providers like you is needed to make a dent in the adverse impact of smoking on health.

The coaching approach to smoking cessation focuses on identifying and changing behaviors and thoughts that keep people smoking. As a coach you will address the smokers' beliefs and attitudes about smoking and quiting. You will identify behaviors that promote smoking and replace them with behaviors that are healthier and help fight smoking urges. Negative or self-defeating thoughts will be replaced with more positive or neutral ways of thinking. In short, we will help change negative thoughts and behaviors through goal-oriented techniques.

Before we begin with the training details of a smoking cessastion program, I would like to reveal to you the most motivated group you can maket this service to---- the expectant mom! This person is the most motivated to stop smoking. Women are more likely to quit smoking during pregnancy than at any other time. We have crafted a letter that you can mail to an OB/GYN doctor that asks for a referral relationship. You can find this letter in your free, marketing resource section of the website. We have also devised flyers to display in the waiting rooms of these areas. Your Smoking Cessation Program will take off like a rocket!

Ok, now for the training stuff.

The following are evidence-based steps in offering a smoking cessation program know as the 5 A's:

1. **Ask** if the indiviual smokes.

2. **Advise** the smoker to quit.

3. **Assess** his or her willingness to quit.

4. **Assist** with intervention.

5. **Arrange** for follow-up progress.

    Let's explore each one:

Ask.

Below you will find a brief questionnaire that can help you assess smoking status, level of dependence on nicotine, and the readiness to quit.

74

Quick Assessment of Dependence and Quitting Potential (With Fagerstrom Test of Nicotine Dependence, or FTND)

1. **How much do you smoke?** The higher the number per day, generally the more dependent the smoker.

10 cigarettes per day or less	(0)
11-20	(1)
21-30	(2)
31 or more	(3)

2. **How soon after waking do you have your first cigarette?** Thirty minutes or less = greater dependence. The answer to this question is one of the best single predictors of relapse.

After 60 minutes	(0)
31-60 minutes	(1)
6-30 minutes	(2)
Within 5 minutes	(3)

3. **Do you smoke more frequently during the first hours after awakening than during the rest of the day?** Smokers who are more dependent will generally smoke considerably more during the beginnng of the day in order to quickly increase nicotine levels and reverse the nicotine deprivation that occurs during sleep.

No	(0)
Yes	(1)

4. **Which cigarette would you hate most to give up?** Generally, smokers who look forward the most to their first cigarette of the day are more dependent than those who favor any other cigarette smoked later In the day.

The first one in the morning	(1)
Any other cigarette of the day	(0)

5. **Do you smoke even if you ae so ill that you are in bed most of the day?** An inability to refrain from smoking even during times of illness suggests a high level of dependence.

No	(0)
Yes	(1)

6. **Do you find it difficult to refrain from smoking in places where it is forbidden?** For example at church, on the bus, or in a meeting? More-dependent smokers will report that this is true of them. However, given recent increases in smoking restrictions, more smokers than not might report that nonsmoking places are problematic for them. They are likely have to exert more effort to find a place to smoke than they previously had to.

No	(0)
Yes	(1)

75

Scoring the FTND. Add up the scored items (1-6) and use the following scale.

0-2	Very low dependence
3-4	Low dependence
5	Moderate dependence
6-7	High dependence
8-10	Very high dependence

Note that this scale identifies relative levels of dependence among smokers. Even those with low dependence will likely have difficulty quitting and will need assistance.

Assessment of Quitting Preparation

7. **Have you tried to quit before; if so, how many times?** The greater the number of planned efforts to stop smoking (i.e. serious attempts at quitting), often the less dependent the individual. Move on the following question if the smoker answered "yes" to this question.

If yes: How long did you remain abstinent, and why did you start smoking again? The longer the duration of abstinence during these attempts, the less dependent the individual is. Also, knowing what methods an individual used and how and why he or she relapsed can provide an idea of what approach to take and what to look out for during this attempt to quit.

8. On a scale of 0-10 with 0 being not at all and 10 being extremely, how interested are you right now in quitting? Use the answer to this question to gauge a smoker's initial motivation to quit at this time.

9. In what situations do you enjoy smoking the most? The answer can indicate some key cues that may be problematic. These cues may elicit urges to smoke after they quit.

10. Do others in the home smoke? A smoke-free home is a good predictor of quitting success. Other smokers in the home will need to accommodate the client to increase his or her chances of success.

11. Have you had problems with alcohol or other drugs? Have you had medical or psychiatric problems? The presence of co-morbid conditions presents additional obstacles and impairs quitting ability. In additon, quitting may impact the blood levels and efficacy of medications clients may be taking for these co-morbid conditions, necessitating medical monitoring. Anyone taking medicine for chronic illnesses should tell his or her doctor they are trying to quit smoking, and give the doctor a chance to review their medications.

Use responses to items 7-11 to develop a treatment plan for motivating and preparing the client to quit smoking.

Advise

When advice comes from a person of perceived authority such as yourself, it can have a modest but significant impact on success. The advise should be clear and direct. "*As your RN Health Coach,*

I am telling you that the single most important and positive thing you can do for yourself and your health right now is to quit smoking. I strongly advise you to quit smoking"

Assess Motivation to Quit

We will use the five stages of behavior change to guide us on this one. The main goal behind using this model is to help clients move in a "forward" direction toward the next stage of readiness. Motivational interviewing can be used to help progress through levels 1-3 and get to action. Some time should be spent In preparing the client to quit or increase motivation before the quit date. (see section on M.I.) Here are the stages:

7. Precontemplation: The smoker has no intention of quitting in the near future.

8. Contemplation: They recognize the problem and are seriously considering quitting, but have not commited to any action.

9. Preparation: The smoker intends to quit in the next month. Specific action plans are developed and solutions explored.

10. Action: The client has stopped smoking and has changed behavior and other items to support the quit attempt and prevent relapse.

11. Maintenance: The client is still working to prevent relapse. This phase begins typicallyafter 3-6 months of maintaining full abstinence.

Below are some common reasons smokers give to continue smoking. The material was derived from Perkins, Conklin & Levine, "A Practical Guidebook to the Most Effective Treatments," 2008.

Reason	Response
It's not a good time.	Frankly put, there is no good time to quit. Quitting is going to be difficult, and life commitments and responsibilities are going to intrude. Try asking the smoker, "When would the perfect time be? What are the odds that everything will align so that such a time will ever occur?" Suggest, "I'm not trying to pressure you; I just want you to honestly consider that the perfect time you envision will likely never arise and now is as good a time as any."
I won't be able to concentrate.	Difficulty concentrating is one of the hallmarks of nicotine withdrawal. The smoker might be a good candidate for nicotine replacement therapy (NRT) such as a patch or gum, which can relieve such symptoms. Try offering, "There are several products you can try that have been demonstrated to reduce the difficulty in concentrating *(Continued)*

Reason	Response
	that quitting smoking can bring about. Lets talk about the different options"
I'll miss it too much.	Recognize the truth in this statement:"Of course you'll miss it; you've been smoking for a long time and it's going to be a hard behavior to leave behind." Suggest that the smoker think of healthy rewards to give him or herself for quiting and staying abstinent. He or she should also begin to think about new behaviors that can take the place of smoking. Remind him or her that when new healthy behaviors ae repeated, they can take the place of smoking and come to be more enticing over time.
I'll gain too much weight.	It is a fact that many people gain weight when they quit smoking(on average, 8-10 pounds). The relative importance of this weight gain compared to quitting smoking should be addressed. Explore this, for example by asking, "What would you think if you gained 10 lbs. and were a nonsmoker for the rest of your life?" The health risks of gaining 10 lbs are a fraction of the risks of continuing to smoke. In order to match the negative impact of smoking on the cardiovascular system alone, an individual would have to gain between 80-100 lbs.
It's how I cope with things.	People who do not smoke have just as many things to cope with as those who do. The difference is that smokers have learned to use smoking as their main method of dealing with life's ups and downs. The truth is that smoking actually does nothing physiologically to help a smoker cope, other than relieving withdrawal. The smoker needs to find healthier ways of coping, which may not seem as helpful as smoking at first, but over time will show that smoking is not necessary for coping. Explore these alternatives with each smoker.
It's who I am.	Is smoking truly a necessary identity? Suggest other things that define this person or other interests that the smoker can embrace. Rather than self-identifying as "I am a smoker," what about " I am a painter, a gardener,

78

Reason	Response
	a runner?" Allowing smoking to be a key identifier is a choice. Encourage the smoker to choose other identities. Ask why he or she cannot identify as a nonsmoker. Potentially, these will be identities which can make the individual feel more proud.
I've tried and failed.	Remind the smoker that he or she is not alone in this regard. Some people try to quit upwards of 15 times before they become nonsmokers for good. Find out what caused difficulty the last time or previous times, and suggest alternative methods of quitting and ways of preparing for trouble spots this time around.

Attacking Ambivalence

Have the smoker develop a list of reasons to quit, followed by a list of reasons to keep smoking. Reasons to quit list:

- Develop positive benefits of quitting. Keep the list framed in the positive. After the list, have the client consider their reasons and explore how quitting achieves each one.

- Have them circle the most important reason for quitting right now. Have the client write a statement about their number one reason and carry it in a pocket to glance at, when an urge arises.

Reasons to continue smoking list:

The client's reasons to continue smoking are just as important. With this list, explore how continuing to smoke achieves the items listed, but unlike the reasons to quit list, these need to be refuted and alternative and healthier strategies to achieve these effects need to be identified. Use the previous chart to help aid in common concerns.

Increasing Motivation

1. inform smokers about the health benefits and risks associated with quitting and continuing to smoke.

2. Explore means of gaining social support. Let others know.

3. increase self-confidence, confidence in the ability to quit.

Some smokers find it motivating to set up a "fun" account to which they contribute a payment for every day of abstinence. This amount should represent a fraction on what they normally spend on smoking. From this account they can reward themselves at the end of the week, or let it build up for that special gift.

A great exercise or something you can do for your client is visit the following website: http://-cancercontrol.cancer.gov/tcrb/smokersrisk/current_smoker.asp

79

This allows smokers to calculate their risk of mortality based on age, smoking rate, years smoking, etc. It shows the impact of smoking on their life expectancy and morbidity. This can be a great motivator. You can also search online for terms such as "smokers' life expectancy calculator" for additional tools.

Potential triggers

Potential triggers for smoking should be assessed and determined prior to the quit date. Preparing for those triggers and deciding beforehand how to deal with them will aid you and the client during the attempt. The most common triggers are paraphernalia associated with smoking. Cigarettes, ashtrays, lighters and matches are strong cues for smoking and should be disgarded prior to quit date. Stay away from smokers. Triggers can be objects, people, places or even moods. Deal with triggers by removing objects, changing routines, avoiding places, and planning to deal with other smokers. A great way to remember how to motivate clients is "**The Five R's.**"

This can also be used as a way to present information or guide conversation

1. **Relevance:** Explore reasons to quit and and reasons to continue. Refute the latter.

2. **Risks:** Provide information on the negative health consequences of smoking.

3. **Rewards:** Explore personal and financial rewards to be gained.

4. **Roadblocks:** Help identify roadblocks and how to deal with them.

5. **Repetition: Review each of the previous four points at every session.**

   Following the above formula will give you a guideline on how to conduct every session and interaction with you client.

Assist with intervention

- Setting a quit date.
- Offer quit date reminders.
- Keep your #1 reason card handy.
- Five R's - continue to motivate the client during every session.
- Coaching along with pharmacotherapy offers the most success.
- Remove or avoid smoking triggers.
- Set strategies for coping with urges or withdrawal.

Quit date

- Quit date should be no more than 2 weeks away when set.
- Consider holiday, weekend, birthday, vacation or anniversary for quit date.
- Prior to date, remind client of upcoming day. Suggest preparation techniques, which have been discussed prior to this. Consider any new ideas.

80

- Consider having client fill out and sign a quitting contract indicating the exact date (see example below).
- Consider a "quitting ceremony" on this day. If you host the ceremony this can be a great marketing and promotional tool for your coaching practice!!

Qutting smoking is the best thing I can do for my health, as well as for the health of those close to me. I have decided that it is time for me to quit for good.

Therefore, I, _____, will quit smoking on _____

_____

My main reasons for quitting smoking include:

_____

_____

_____

_____

I know that quitting will have the following positive benefits:

_____

_____

_____

_____

The worst things about smoking that I will be happy to be rid of include:

_____

_____

_____

_____

One person who I can contact for support while I work to stay away from cigarettes is:

_____

_____   _____
Signature   Date

_____   _____
Witness Signature   Date

81

Make sure the above contract has your contact, logo, signage, etc.

Present this to client on high-grade paper and framed.

More on handling triggers

Be aware that most urges only last a few minutes and the desire will pass with time. The urges will pass even more quickly if smokers have a specific strategy for coping. Consider the following:

- Cognitive strategies: reminder of positive conequences. Have #1 reason handy.
- Stay busy: puzzles, books, walks, movies, visiting friends.
- Keep hands active: holding items, pencil, straw, stress ball (branded of course with your company info).
- Have healthy snacks at hand and chewing gum.
- Relaxation techniques.

What if a smoker can t abstain right away?

For those and only those having a difficult time quitting right away, try either of these two intermediate steps:

1. Scheduled reduction.
2. Narrowing the smoking environment.

it is important to remember the ultimate goal is still abstinence.

Schedule reduction

Schedule reduction Involves systematically reducing the amount of smoking over time, by gradually lengthening the time between each cigarette. This forces the smoker to cope with cravings to smoke that occur before it is time for the next cigarette. Initially, the schedule can include the same number of cigarettes per day a smoker usually smokes. So, if a smoker smokes 25 cigarettes per day, they can be instructed to smoke one cigarette every 40 minutes (assuming they are awake for 16-17hrs/day).

What generally happens is, the smoker loses track of time and allows more than 40 mintues to pass before realizing it. This should tell the smoker that they have the ability to prevent cravings by engaging in coping strategies, such as staying busy. The smoker cannot have another smoke until the next authorized time. The number of cigarettes allowed per day or time interval should be changed fairly rapidly, at least every week if not more frequently. Each reduction should be in steps of 5 or so - 25/day, down to 20/day, to 15 and so on.

Narrowing smoking locations

Narrowing smoking locations means placing limits on when and where the smokers allows himself or herself to smoke. The smoker should choose only one or two places where he or she allows himself or herself to smoke. The smoker should also select locations that are undesirable and not where they

82

would otherwise want to stay. The smoker is no longer allowed to smoke in his or her normal locations, only 1- 2 unpleasant ones, such as a metal chair in the garage or dumpster outside of work.

Medications to Aid the quitting process

Why coaching is still needed and to used along with medications

1. Explain limitations of medications.
2. Explain how to use the medications.
3. Help adjust to the end of medication use.

First-line medications for quitting smoking. FDA approved.

1. Nicotine Replacement Therapy (NRT)
2. Bupropion or Zyban
3. Carenicline or Chantix

NRT

A common, but false belief, is that nicotine is the chief villian in the adverse health effects of smoking. While nicotine is what causes people to become addicted or dependent on smoking, it is the other chemicals that are responsible for the damaging health effects, especially cancer. This is important to understand, so that the safety of nicotine replacement therapy can be recognized.

The rapid speed of nicotine delivery by smoking explains the addictiveness of tobacco smoking vs. NRT, which delivers nicotine more slowly and is far less addictive. NRT has a low potential for causing addiction because of the speed and route.

NRT is based on the principle that replacing the nicotine delivered by smoking using a safer method of delivery will lessen the severity of withdrawal and craving. The replacement of nicotine without introducing any other harmful ingredients is made.

Although NRT should be used in all populaions, it should be noted that women tend to have a poorer response to NRT than men.

Nicotine Patch

In formal clinical trails that included counseling and the patch, approximately 20%-25% of the patients were not smoking at 6 months, vs. 10% for the placebo patch (Fiore,Smith,Jorenby,&Baker,1994).

Nicotine Gum

Speed of delivery is quicker than the patch, but still slower than smoking.

Nasal spray & Inhaler

These two are only offered with a prescription from a doctor.

Nicotine Lozenge

Smokeless Cigarettes

Although these products are not FDA approved for smoking cessation, your clients may benefit from the satisfaction of the oral route for delivery, as well as the nicotine replacement. You can also distribute and sell this product yourself to add a new source of income to your coaching business. Check out www.StopSmokingHealthCoach.com for more information.

Prescription Meds

Bupropion/Zyban/Wellbutrin

Clinical trails show that the use of this medication doubles the success rate compared to placebo, 30-35% vs. 15% (Fioreet al., 2000; Hurt et al.,1997).

The most common side effect is insomnia(about 30%).

The medication may also limit weight gain that occurs after quitting.

Therapeutic blood levels should be achieved prior to quit date, therefore dosing should begin 1-2 weeks before the quit date, and continued 7-12 weeks following the quit date.

Varenicline/Chantix

A newer drug. Clinical trials show superior quit rates than with bupropion or placebo. 30% for varenicline, 23% for bupropion and 15-17% for placebo (Gonzales et al., 2006; Jorenby et al., 2006).

Nausea may occur in about 30%. Treatment should begin 1 week prior to quit date.

Arrange for follow up

Phone calls should be scheduled in advance to avoid any phone tag.

Determine the agenda ahead of time and be upfront about the purpose of the call and how long the call will last. You might tell the caller you will call once a week, for x minutes and the purpose will be to:

- determine progress.
- assess craving and withdrawal.
- review medication usage or reactions.
- review coping techniques.
- discuss any other difficulties the client is having and briefly problem solve.
- offer encouragement.
- remind when the next call or visit is.

If it is determined that a client is having a difficult time, you may want to suggest an additional session be scheduled.

Withdrawal & Lapses

Signs and symptoms of withdrawal will begin within 2 hours of the last nicotine use. These symptoms may peak within 24-48 hours after quiting and last anywhere from a few days to several weeks. The use of NRT will help with the withdrawal effects. Provide the greatest support during the first 24-48 hours and remind the client that withdrawal is a temporary condition.

Several scales can be used to assess wihdrawal. See www.uvm.edu/~hbpl/?page=minnesota/-default.html

If a client slips up and has a smoke, this is called a lapse. If they return to regular smoking, this is a relapse. If they have a smoke, let them know that this lapse does not have to become a relapse. At this point they should review the situation that led to the lapse and make an immediate recovery plan. Clients often lapse because of the situation and how they coped or did not cope with the triggers that presented, not because they are weak-willed. Go over the situation and reformulate the plan. A typical response to a lapse should be something like: *"It sounds like you had a slip in smoking. This is called a lapse and the fact that we are talking about it rather than you returning to smoking is impressive and shows your comittment to quiting. You haven't blown it, the slip is behind us now and you are still a non-smoker, but you need to recommit to staying that way. Tell me about the events leading up to the slip"*

Smoking and weight Concerns

Smokers typically weigh less than non-smokers. Almost all smokers will gain some weight when they quit. The average weight gain is about 8 -10 pounds over the following year, with most occuring in the first month.

As a smoking cessation coach, the most effective stategy is to work on changing the attitudes about weight gain related to quitting rather than attacking the weight gain itself. The health benefits of not smoking far outweigh the health effects of a modest weight gain followed by quitting tabacco use. Be sure you remind the client of this. An ex-smoker would need to gain in excess of 80 pounds to negate the health benefits of quitting.

How smoking affects weight

Smoking affects both sides of the energy balance equation, both calorie Intake and calorie expenditure.

On the intake side, smokers tend to eat less snacks between meals. Their food consumption is lowered because smoking enhances and prolongs the feeling of satiety or fullness after meals.

On the expenditure side, which relates to tho body's resting metabolic rate and amount of physical activity, smoking increases the resting metabolism.

Dieting during smoking cessation efforts may be counterproductive and is not advised until about 6-12 months of being smoke free. Weight loss and smoking cessation are separate and difficult health behaviors that should be approached one at a time, starting with smoking, which is the most critical one.

85

Smoking Resources

www.cgtri.wisc.edu/HC.Providers/healthcare.htm
contains links to provider training materials

www.aptna.org/APTNA_Resources.html
slides and handouts on starting a cessation program

www.surgeongeneral.gov/tobacco/
materials for both clients and coaches

www.smokeclinic.com/home.asp
materials for clients and coaches

www.trytostop.org
create personalized quit plans and quit calendars
smoking resources

www.becomeanex.org/core/whatisex.aspx
resources for coaches
personalized plans for smokers

www.smokefree.gov
interactive site to determine personal risk: http://smokefree.gov/smokersrisk/
resources relevant to different steps in quitting process

www.lungusa.com
free online Freedom From Smoking cessation program broken up into self-paced modules

Worksite Wellness

Rising healthcare costs are a great concern to American business. The costs continue to rise about twice as fast as general inflation. If no action is taken, expectations of 6-12% increase a year are inevitable. A lot of this cost has been transferred to the employees, who pay about 16% of premiums for individuals and 27% for families. As a result of this trend, both businesses and employees should be motivated to keep healthcare costs as low as possible. Generally healthy and fit employees have lower health care costs. Worksite wellness is a solution!

What Employers Want To Do

- Control High Health Care Cost
- Retain Good Workers
- Attract Good Employees
- Improve Productivity
- Improve Employee Morale
- Improve Corporate Image

What Employees Want Access To

- Screenings for high risk conditions
- Disease prevention
- Longer life
- Higher quality of life
- A way to feel better and have more energy
- A way to lose weight
- A way to decrease personal health cost

Controlling high health care costs

The U.S. is the top spender on health per capita. Health care costs account for 16% of our GDP in recent years. Our spending on healthcare has been increasing 2-5 times the rate of inflation since 2000.

Research shows that healthcare costs are tied to risk factors and health practices. Generally healthy, fit employees have lower health care costs.

Obesity and Healthcare Costs

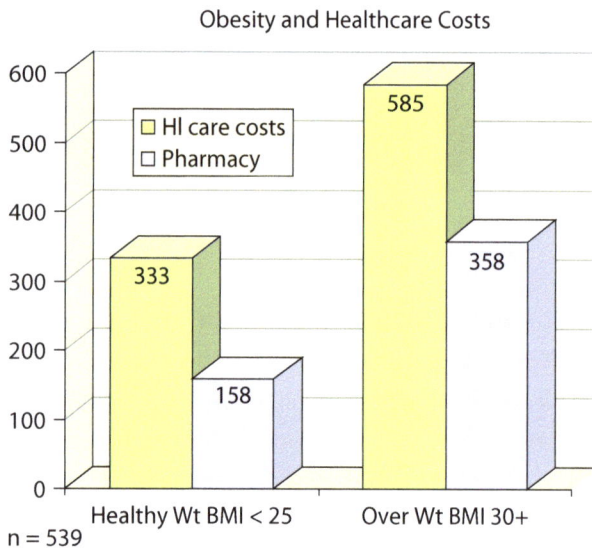

n = 539

Median annual health care costs were 75% higher ($252) in the over-weight group compared to the healthy weight group.

Kaiser Permanente Study, Archives of Internal Medicine, Oct. 25, 2004

Individuals with unhealthy BMI's are 3.8 times more likely to be hospitalized and 2-3 times more likely to have outpatient visits.

GM Study – Overweight and Healthcare Costs

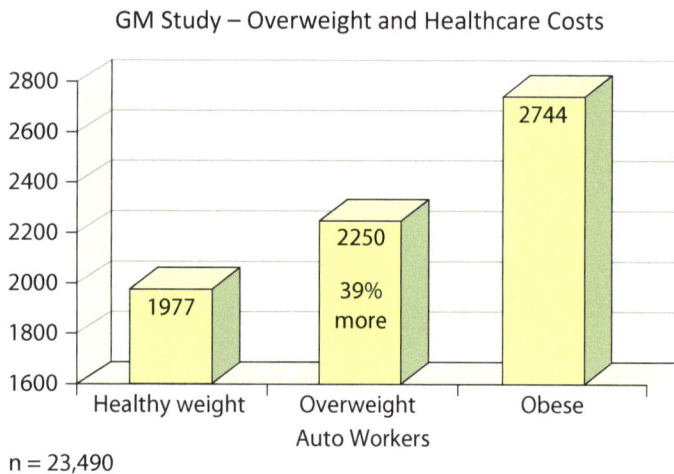

n = 23,490

- **Overweight workers cost $273 more/yr than healthy weight workers.**
- **Obese workers (BMI 30+) cost $767 more per year than normal weight active employees.**

Source: Journal of Occupational and Environmental Medicine, May 2004

Improving Productivity

When employees are physically and mentally healthy, they are more likely to be on the job and performing well.

According to M. O'Donnell, writing in the American Journal of Health Promotion, health promotion activities are likely to yield greater returns from increased productivity than from medical care cost savings.

Each additional risk factor an employee has is associated with a 2.4% decrease in productivity.**

88

The full cost of injury and illness

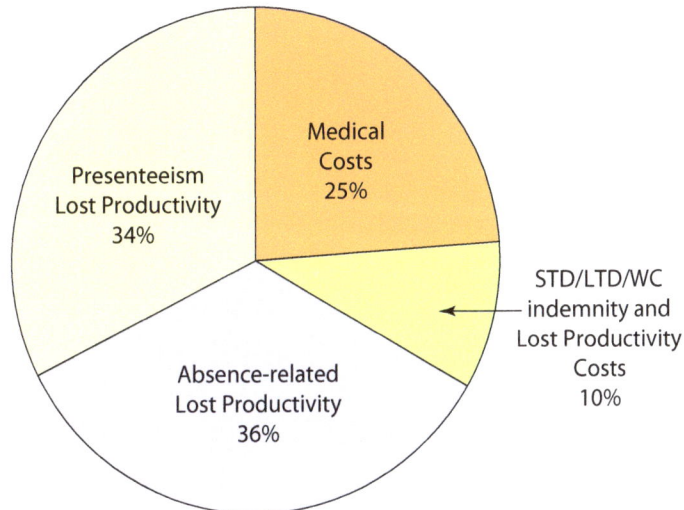

Adapted from: Integrated Benefits Institute: May 2007

To reduce absenteeism and disability

Such items as back injuries are very common in the overweight and unfit workers. This can represent a major cause of work loss time and disability which is very costly.

> **"Companies with the most effective health and productivity programs experienced superior performance in three significant areas:**
>
> - **Achieved 20 percent more revenue per employee**
> - **Have 16.1 percent higher market value**
> - **Delivered 57 percent higher shareholder returns."**
>
> **Building an Effective Health & Productivity Framework 2007/2008 Staying@Work Report, Watson Wyatt Worldwide**

1. Make the above argument, gain support of decision maker.
2. Plan & discuss budget.
3. Perform HRA.
4. Perform Culture Survey.
5. Plan interventions / Programs.
   A. Life Style Management /Health Coaching

      Condition-Specific Weight Loss

8 Weeks to wellness

Smoking Cessation

Emotional Health & Mind Body

(Any other program you may design)

B. Disease Management

Diabetes

Hypertension

CHD

Cancer

C. Newsletters

D. Self-study

E. Screenings

F. Seminars "lunch and learns"

G. Incentive programs

Marketing

Currently 62% of larger companies with greater than 200 employees are offering wellness programs. 26% of companies with less than 200 employees are offering wellness programs

-Look for small businesses in the range of 100-1000 employees.

-Build in a 20-30% margin in your price. Ask for performance-based pay.

HRA

Conducting a Health Risk Assessment will allow you to identify risks and interests of the employees, allowing you to decide on which programs to offer. It is the foundation for measuring and evaluating changes and or improvements from year to year.

Average participation rates for HRA are around 30% for year 1, reaching a cumulative participation rate of 70% at year 6. A 70% participation rate is needed to achieve an impact. The greatest participation can be achieved by implementing incentives along with the HRA.

HRA categories of risk:

Low risk 0-2

Medium risk 3-4

High risk 5+

Existing disease - offer disease-management programs or referrals.

High risk - offer risk-reduction programs such as health coaching.

Low risk - offer health-promotion programs to prevent high risks, such as newsletters, self study or seminars.

http://www.hmrc.umich.edu/research/cost-ben.html

Composition of an average company

Source: Journal of Occupational & Environmental Medicine. Vol 47(8): 769-777.
The below represents the average risk in companies.

0 risk 15%

1 risk 28%

2-3 risk 43%

4-5 risks 12%

6+ risks 2%

http://www.hmrc.umich.edu/research/steelcase.html

Budget:

Research shows that an investment of anywhere from $150-$400 per employee is needed to yield a positive Return on Investment for wellness programs. When talking to decision makers, instead of asking for a specific dollar amount, ask for a percentage of the employee's entire benefit package to equal $150-$400. For example, if an employee's entire benefits package is $4,000, ask for 1% of the benefits package to be used for wellness, which is $100 in this case.

The range in fees comes from the different types of programs. Awareness and supportive environment programs are much cheaper than behavior change programs.

See your resource disk for a sample budget template.

ROI (Return On Investment)

Companies that do not run a comprehensive wellness program generally will not see a positive ROI. It is not enough to hold an annual health fair, host an occasional class or provide literature without follow up. When a comprehensive program is in place ROI's of greater than 3:1 are seen after the 3rd year.

Incentives:

Should be meaningful, memorable and measurable.

Limitation on reward should not exceed 20% of cost of health plan.

See HIPA final wellness regulations: 71Fed. Reg 7514.

Help employee see perceived value. For example, testing service value $190, paid for by your em-

91

ployer, good for 30 days.

Programs that use incentives have higher overall participation.

Approximately 2/3 of all employers offer an incentive.

Assessing Corporate Culture

An assessment should be made of the corporate culture. Efforts can be made to improve the wellness culture through providing a healthy work environment, creating a budget for wellness. Here are some policies and practices:

- Offer healthy food choices in cafeteria and healthy snacks in vending machines.
- Start a non-smoking policy.
- Provide only healthy foods at meetings.
- Develop a wellness committee.
- Provide an annual health screening and HRA.
- Offer incentives for participating in wellness.

Conclusion

As risks come down, so will cost! Employers can take a reactive approach to healthcare, continue to pay for problems after they occur, and watch costs skyrocket, or they can take the pro-active approach, where they invest in the health and wellness of their employees and lower healthcare cost and improve productivity.

Conclusions

RN Health Coaching offers a tremendous opportunity to use your skills to resolve one of the fastest-rising conditions in the country; obesity and its related effects. The work you do can dramatically improve quality of life, quality of health and length of life. You can use your skills to improve your income, advance your personal goals and save lives.

92

Resources

Health Care Insurance Cost
http://www.nchc.org/facts/cost.shtml

Wellness & Health Promotion Organizations
American Journal of Health
www.healthpromotionjournal.com

Wellness Councils of America
www.welcoa.org

Wellness Councils of Canada
www.welcan.com

National Wellness Institute
www.nationalwellness.org

Government Resources
1. National Center for Chronic Disease Prevention & Health Promotion, Centers for Disease Control and Prevention
www.cdc.gov

National Heart, Lung & Blood Institute
www.nhlbi.nih.gov

National Health Information Center
www.health.gov/nhic/

Office of Disease Prevention & Health Promotion
http://odphp.osophs.dhhs.gov

Weight Information Network
www.Win.niddk.nih.gov

National Institutes of Health
www.nih.gov

Nutrition
US Department of Agriculture
www.usda.gov

Disease
National Cancer Institute
www.nci.nih.gov

93

Notes

[i]Domrose, Cathryn, **NurseWeek,** April 30, 2002, Online 1/11/09 @: http://www.nurseweek.com/news/features/02-04/future.asp

[ii]The American Heart Association: Heart Disease & Stroke Statistics 2008 Update at a Glance, American Heart Association: Online 1/11/09 @ http://americanheart.org/downloadable/heart/1200078608862HS_Stats%202008.final.pdf

[iii]Ibid.

[iv]Wang, Beydoun, Liang, et. Al., Obesity: A Research Journal, (2008) 16, 10, 2323-2330

[v]US Department of Health and Human Services, National Institutes of Health, Obesity Threatens to Cut US Life Expectancy, New Analysis Suggests, March 16, 2005, Online 1/11/09 @ http://www.nih.gov/news/pr/mar2005/nia-16.htm

[vi]Ibid.

[vii]Bio-Medicine, Online 1/11/09 @ http://www.bio-medicine.org/medicine-news/Dietary-Counseling-Leads-to-Weight-Loss-23807-1/

[viii]Arloski, Michael, Ph.D., Wellness Coaching for Lasting Lifestyle Change, Whole Person Associates Publishing, Duluth, MN, pg. 13.

[ix]Fierce Healthcare: Daily News for Healthcare Executives: Trend: Health Coach Popularity keeps Growing, November 19, 2006, Online 1/23/09 @ http://www.fiercehealthcare.com/story/trend-health-coach-popularity-keeps-growing/2006-11-20

[x]WATKO Benefit Group, Health Coaches help Workers, Save Companies Cash, Online 1/23/09 @ http://www.watkobenefit.com/s/700/index.aspx?sid=700&gid=1&pgid=252&cid=847&ecid=847&crid=0&calpgid=304&calcid=823

[xii]Arloski, Michael, Ph.D., Wellness Coaching for Lasting Lifestyle Change, Whole Person Associates Publishing, Duluth, MN, pg. 62.

[xiii]Health Coaching UK: Benefits for Business: Boost Productivity with a Happy Well Motivated Work Force, Online 1/28/09 @ http://www.healthcoachinguk.com/page4.htm

[xiv]Schroeder, Debbie, How Health Coaching Leads to Permanent Weight Loss, Self Growth.com, Online 1/29/09 @ http://www.selfgrowth.com/articles/How_Health_Coaching_Leads_to_Permanent_Weight_Loss.html

[xv]The Coaching Starter Kit: Everything You Need to Launch and Expand Your Coaching Practice, Coachville.com, W.W. Norton, New York, 2003, pg. 19.

[xvi]Arloski, Michael, Ph.D., Wellness Coaching for Lasting Lifestyle Change, Whole Person Associates Publishing, Duluth, MN, pgs. 42-48.

[xvi]Arloski, Michael, Ph.D., Wellness Coaching for Lasting Lifestyle Change, Whole Person Associates Publishing, Duluth, MN, pg. 4.

** Journal of Occupational & Environmental Medicine 47(8):769-777

* Kaiser Permanente study, achieves of internal Medicine

While Dwayne Adams has been an active and successful registered nurse for over a decade, working in critical care and other areas of the field, he is also an accomplished entrepreneur. Capitalizing on his nursing expertise, he combined it with his business skills to create a successful new enterprise.

Along with his nursing education, Adams earned a bachelor's degree in business administration in the area of marketing, as well as a master's degree in finance. This education outside of the nursing field has given him the added edge he needed in order to become a successful entrepreneur and lead his companies from growth through expansion.

His first business-related endeavor was to bridge the gap between registered nurses and those who could benefit from working with a health and wellness coach. With this idea in mind, he created a whole new concept and coined the term "RN Health Coach." His business concept of registered nurses becoming health coaches has been well received, and many nurses around the country have followed his lead and benefited from his advice.

As a business-savvy registered nurse, Adams not only created a lucrative new career field for those in nursing, but has also used his skills, education and experience to help them to be successful entrepreneurs. He understands what it takes to build a business, market it, and sustain it long-term.

Given the state of health that people across the nation are currently in, Adams has shown his genius by creating the RN Heath Coach field. His passion for helping nurses to put their skills and education to use beyond the setting of a hospital bedside, combined with his entrepreneurial mindset, has created a lucrative field for registered nurses to enter.

He has developed a recipe for success that creates a win-win situation for all involved. Registered nurses get the pleasure of doing what they love – helping people – while those in the community who need health and wellness coaching get the most qualified coaches available.

Adams has a unique perspective on the business world, because of his nursing background. This allows him to actively pinpoint the most effective ways for RN Health Coaches to build, promote, and enjoy their new career field. He is an expert in the areas of nursing and health and wellness coaching, but also in marketing, finance, and business. Visit him at www.TheNurseExpert.com

95

SUGGESTED BOOK TITLES

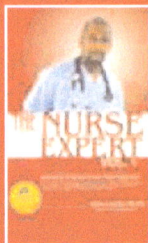

The Nurse Expert vol. 1
Secrets to being your own publicist.
ISBN: 978-0-9850033-1-9

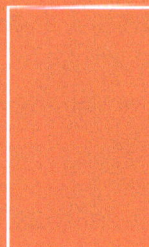

The Nurse Expert vol. 3
Your 3 Step formula for success.
ISBN: 978-0-9850033-2-6

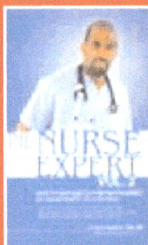

The Nurse Expert vol. 2
How to use radio to position yourself as
the authority in your field.
ISBN: 978-0-9850033-0-2

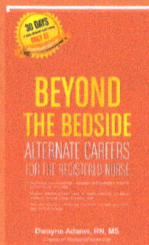

Beyond The Bedside,
Alternative Careers for Nurses.
ISBN: 978-0-9850033-3-3

TheNurseExpert.com